Therapy and Consultation in Child Care

Therapy in Child Care and *Consultation in Child Care* are two classics of clinical and theoretical work on psychotherapy with severely disturbed children. Residential psychotherapeutic communities based on Barbara Dockar-Drysdale's principles have unrivalled reputations for success with the kind of young offenders who are most likely to become lifelong re-offenders. The young people who have been in her care have astonishingly low rates of re-offending.

The author is Britain's leading figure in this field. She worked closely with Donald Winnicott in the period after World War Two and applied his ideas, while developing her own, to children so damaged that it was often felt that they could not be helped. Her method is covered here in depth, and focused on initiating and strengthening a process of repair in the child, enabling a cycle of anti-social or criminal behaviour to be broken.

The books are reprinted by popular demand from workers in the field at a time when those who care for the social fabric are shocked by the dreadful things that some young people do. The principles espoused in this book are the humane alternative to the 'get tough' approach usually adopted by governments, or in the face of moral panics.

BARBARA DOCKAR-DRYSDALE founded and was director of the Mulberry Bush School. She went on to become Consultant Psychotherapist to the Cotswold Community in Gloucestershire. She is the author of *The Provision of Primary Experience: Winnicottian Work with Children and Adolescents* (Free Association Books, 1990).

Therapy and Consultation in Child Care

Barbara Dockar-Drysdale

Foreword by D. W. Winnicott

'an association in which the free development of each
is the condition of the free development of all'

Free Association Books / London / 1993

Therapy and Consultation in Child Care
first published in Great Britain in 1993 by
Free Association Books Ltd
26 Freegrove Road
London N7 9RQ

The publication of
Therapy and Consultation in Child Care
was aided by generous support from the
Planned Environment Therapy Trust.

Therapy in Child Care first published as Volume 3 of
Longman Papers on Residential Work
© Longman Group Ltd, 1968

Consultation in Child Care first published as Volume 4 of
Longman Papers on Residential Work
© Longman Group Ltd, 1973

ISBN 1 85343 194 X

A CIP catalogue record for this book is available
from the British Library.

Printed in the EC

Therapy in Child Care

To my husband

Contents

Foreword

This collection of papers speaks for itself. I do welcome the chance, however, to assist at the launching of a book that I feel sure will be of value to those who are engaged in residential work with children.

When I first met Mrs Dockar-Drysdale I was excited to find someone who was receptive in an active way. So often one feels: if you don't know, how can I tell you! Here was someone who knew, and who therefore enriched what she heard. On the basis of a wide experience of the actual care of well and ill children she was developing into a sophisticated therapist and conceptualizer. Now she has certainly reached the stage at which she can use her accumulated experience in order to hand on ideas to those doing similar work who want to think about their work.

A good example of Mrs Dockar-Drysdale's contribution comes from her use of the term *frozen child*. The alternative term *affectionless child* has proved to be a useful clinical description, but the term *frozen child* gives us the defence organization that has value to the child in that it brings invulnerability, an idea which carries with it the idea of potential suffering. Also, the nickname *archipelago child* catches on better than the terms unintegrated, disintegrated, de-integrated, as an apt clinical description of an easily recognized type of case in which six people meet a child and seem to see six different children.

Also I admire Mrs Dockar-Drysdale's handling of the idea of *the survival of the therapist* as an important factor, along with the need for the inanimate objects to be not *too well* protected, so that the child may be able to do *some* damage, and reach to a personal urge to make restitution.

Finally, the idea of *primary experience* seems to me to be well named and its use well defined, and its relation to the psycho-analytic concept of transference usefully discussed. One can see easily from these pages that the provision of primary experience is fundamental to the therapy of children who have been let down in infancy or earliest childhood.

I have learned much from Mrs Dockar-Drysdale; in writing this preface I wish to express my personal gratitude for work she had done with my patients, and also for ideas that she has given me or has made significant by using in the practice of residential care and therapy.

D. W. Winnicott

Acknowledgements

We are grateful to the following for permission to reproduce the undermentioned previously published articles by Mrs Dockar-Drysdale:

Association of Psychiatric Social Workers for 'Outsiders and insiders in a therapeutic school' from *Boundaries of Casework*; the Editor of *The British Journal of Criminology* for 'Some aspects of damage and restitution' (1953) and 'The residential treatment of "frozen" children' (1958) from *The British Journal of Delinquency*; The Howard League for Penal Reform for 'Communication as a technique in treating disturbed children' (1959) from *The Howard Journal*; North-Holland Publishing Company for 'Notes on the history of the development of a projection technique' from *Acta Psychologica*; *The New Era* for 'Notes on selection' (1960) and 'The process of symbolization observed among emotionally deprived children' (1962); and Pergamon Press Ltd. for 'The provision of primary experience' (1966) from *The Journal of Child Psychology and Psychiatry*.

Permission has also been kindly granted for the following quotations:

From *The Psychoanalytical Review*, New York, for the quotation from Lili E. Peller's paper 'Libidinal development as reflected in play' on pages 135–6; from Virginia M. Axline and her publishers the Houghton Mifflin Company, Boston, for the eight principles of play out of 'Play therapy' quoted on pages 142–6; from Professor Erik H. Erikson and W. W. Norton and Company Inc., New York, for the quotation from 'Childhood and Society' on page 155.

The Mulberry Bush School

The background to the problems concerning the residential treatment of disturbed children, which are discussed in this collection of papers, was the Mulberry Bush School. In common with several other therapeutic ventures it put down roots during the period of evacuation from London, towards the end of World War II. My husband was serving in the Middle East, while I lived in a house near his family home in Berkshire. I started a small play group for our own and neighbourhood children, in a friend's house; we called it 'the Mulberry Bush' because this house had a mulberry tree in the garden. When the play group evolved later into a nursery school in our own home we kept the name 'the Mulberry Bush'. At that time there were many mothers and children in difficulties caused by wartime conditions, so that soon we collected several mothers and their children to live with us in addition to our own family.

During this phase of development I met Milan Morgenstern, an Austrian psychotherapist who had come as a refugee from Nazi Germany to live in our neighbourhood, and it was thanks to him that I first read Freud (in German).

One day I was asked to provide a holiday for an unhappy little boy. I was so worried about him that I wrote a report for the social worker who had sent Pat to us. This report started a chain of circumstances which led to a visit from Dr Dingwell (an educational psychologist, at that time working for the National Association of Mental Health). She was very interested in what I was trying to do for the mothers and children in our house, and took matters further; so that presently we were visited by representatives of the Ministry of Education. These people were deeply concerned with the provision of treatment for the many disturbed children whose problems had first been brought to light by evacuation. As a result of this visit and the discussion which took place that day, the Ministry of Education suggested that I should find a suitable house which was large enough for a school for maladjusted children. Here I could develop my ideas and put them into practice with some financial support (with fees approved by the Ministry under Section 91 of the Education Act of 1944). The Berkshire Education Authority offered school medical care; and was unstinting in help and advice, which was much needed in every way. In fact, from the start of the Mulberry Bush until the present time, we have continued to receive teaching and help from many sources, especially from child psychiatrists, psychologists and psychiatric social workers; without whose generous help the Mulberry Bush could never have survived. We continue to work very closely with Child Guidance clinics.

In the spring of 1948 my husband was demobilized: he returned to a maelstrom of activity, into which he plunged practically, emotionally, and economically. The house at Standlake (which I had found through personal contacts) was bought entirely thanks to him, and he gave up an appointment in the Ministry of Food in order to help me to establish the school, in which we were to work together for fifteen years.

The papers which I have collected are nearly all concerned with work carried out in the Mulberry Bush from 1948 to 1963. During these years I underwent a personal analysis (Freudian), which was necessary and valuable in my work with children and staff. My analysis taught me an emotional economy which has stood me in good stead. During this period the school passed through all sorts of difficulties: during its early days the way in which we worked seemed alien to many people, and for some time we felt rather isolated. Some of my first papers were written in an attempt to come out of this isolation. The establishment of the Association of Workers for Maladjusted Children (of which we were among the first members) brought the Mulberry Bush into contact with other schools also doing experimental work; thus our isolation ended. We came to know people in our own particular field, many of whom have given advice and encouragement. I would like especially to thank Dr Marjorie Franklin, Father Owen, Otto

Shaw and David Wills, all of whom have made such important contributions to residential treatment, and are so concerned for people working in schools for maladjusted children.

The description of the school which follows refers to the first twelve years of its existence, and was written during that period.

The school is a non-profit-making limited company, run by a Board of Directors and fully recognized by the Ministry of Education. From the very beginning we have selected only deeply disturbed children, of average intelligence, in the age range of five to twelve years. There were, at the time I am describing, forty children and twenty-three adults. The aim of treatment was to return the children to normal life as soon as possible; or, in the case of deprived children, to a children's home, foster home, or whatever seemed suitable. The average length of stay was two years.

There were four lesson groups, ranging from the 'smalls', a group which had little structure but provided early educational experience; to the 'bigs', where there was a very definite structure, formal education, and from which children usually returned to more normal school life. These were the planned groups: there were also, of course, the spontaneous groups; these evolved during what Bettelheim (1950) calls 'in-between times'—before and after meals, during school play times, in the evenings and at weekends. Because of the way in which treatment was carried out, a deep bond was usually established between lesson group and teacher; it was then possible for this bond to come into all fields of the children's lives in the school. The team worked closely together with a great deal of mutual support, and there was also steady support from outside from our directors and from referring child guidance clinics. Psychiatrists supervised treatment of the children they sent to us, while psychiatric social workers helped the parents, and also ourselves in our work with parents (who visited their children frequently).

My husband and I were co-principals. He established and supported the therapeutic environment, planning administration in a way that left me free to supervise and carry out therapeutic work within the school, and to maintain close liason with parents and referring clinics. Had it not been for his support none of us could have tolerated the strain of the particular work we did. The need for a very special kind of paternal support was essential.

There was a head teacher and three other teachers; a domestic bursar, a matron and a deputy matron. This was the treatment team. There was also the cook-housekeeper, the school secretary, and a large domestic staff; all were in touch with both team and children.

In 1959 the Mulberry Bush was recognized by the Ministry of Education and became a non-profit-making company run by a Board of Directors. This change brought many advantages and some unforeseen difficulties: the management of a therapeutic school presents very great problems, with which our committee continues to strive to this day. This school, as our directors of course realize, is more like a living organism than an institutional organization: to evolve a flexible yet practical and economic administration involves labours worthy of Hercules. There have been times of great stress and anxiety for both management and team, during these years, but out of the difficulties has emerged a therapeutic organization, in every area of which the provision of primary experience for emotionally deprived children remains the basic task.

The school was reorganized about six years ago. My husband withdrew in order to take up work of his own. Without his long and devoted service to the school it could not have continued its existence. A headmaster was appointed, and I continued to work part-time in the school as therapeutic adviser. I was by now a psychotherapist and a member of the Association of Psychotherapists.

I cannot here acknowledge all my innumerable debts to the many people who have helped me. It will be evident how much I owe to Dr D. W. Winnicott, with whom I have been able to discuss my work for many years, and who has supported me through many difficulties. My husband and my children have all faced the hazards of life in and about a therapeutic school: without their love and encouragement I would not have lived long enough to write these papers! Several generations of Mulberry Bush teams have worked far beyond their capacity to give therapeutic help to emotionally deprived children in this special and exacting way: these papers are a record of the work which we have done together. The present headmaster, John Armstrong, and his team are now providing primary experience for emotionally deprived children with deep concern and great skill, using techniques which are based on the ideas expressed in the following papers.

Certain Child Guidance clinics have been referring children to us and helping us through the whole history of the school. I am thinking especially of the Ealing Child Guidance Centre, the East London Child Guidance Clinic, St George's Hospital Clinic, the Paddington Green Clinic, and the Tavistock Clinic. Dr Portia Holman of the Ealing Child Guidance Centre (the founder of the Association of Workers for Maladjusted Children) has always given much help to us, as she has to so many schools for disturbed children. Dr Augusta Bonnard of the East London Clinic has, from the start, been prepared to discuss and clarify problems connected with the work of the Mulberry Bush School. Dr D. W. Winnicott and Dr Barbara Woodhead both worked for many years at Paddington Green Hospital, where conferences have always been enriching experiences. At the Tavistock Clinic it has been in particular the psychiatric social workers who have taught me so much that has been of use to the school; especially Mrs Elizabeth Irvine (who is now Reader in Social Studies at York University).

Dr Edna Oakeshott, who is Senior Lecturer in the education of maladjusted children at the University of London Institute of Education, and Richard Balbernie, who was until recently Research Fellow to the Institute of Education of Bristol University and is now headmaster of the Cotswold Community (an approved school), are two other friends of the school with whom it has always been possible and valuable to discuss my problems and those of the Mulberry Bush.

I am most grateful to Mr Robert Tod, both for his work on the index and for the encouragement and valuable advice which he has given me in the preparation of the book.

There have been many other people who have helped us; and, as will become evident in the course of reading these papers, without such support this sort of work cannot be done.

Finally, I must thank most deeply my secretary, Kate Britton, who has revised and arranged these papers; a complicated task which she has performed with skill and patience.

NOTE

I have arranged my papers chronologically, since all the ideas discussed in this book are based on actual experiences in the course of the history of the Mulberry Bush School and also of myself. Thus 'Context Profiles', one of the later papers in this collection, describes a project carried out by the present headmaster, John Armstrong, and his team.

The reader will notice that I have sometimes used the same clinical material more than once in illustration. I must apologize, but I have been unable to find other equally appropriate material which I could use in these contexts.

References to other papers I have written appear from time to time in the text. Most of such papers are in this volume; but two, 'Symbolization' and 'Adaptation to Individual Needs in a Group' have already been republished in the second volume of Papers on Residential Work.

I

Some aspects of damage and restitution, 1953

During the years 1952 to 1953, Dr Emmanuel Miller allowed me to attend case conferences every Thursday in the department of Psychological Medicine of St George's Hospital. I found these conferences most exciting and stimulating: discussion was invariably very interesting, and therapists were undefended in talking about difficulties as well as successes.

One day Dr Miller suggested that I should read a paper to the team about some aspect of my work at the Mulberry Bush. 'Damage and Restitution' was the first paper I had ever written, and I was anxious and uncertain; but at least I would not be talking to strangers! In fact, the paper met with a warm reception and was followed by a discussion which helped me to gain insight into several problems. Dr Miller asked me to submit this first manuscript to the (then) British Journal of Delinquency, where it was published. I remember that Dr Edward Glover helped me to reconstruct the paper, and gave me invaluable advice.

My choice of subject was important, since I was at that time struggling to communicate my first experiences with emotionally deprived children. I was thankful for Aichhorn's Wayward Youth (1935), but I nevertheless found it difficult to show the justification of a treatment approach which accepted destructive behaviour as often inevitable.

Nowadays I would be talking about annihilation and creation, rather than damage and restitution. I would not now believe that all children are capable at any time of making restitution; I certainly needed to believe this at that stage of my own evolvement. However, there is much in this first paper which links with the work which we do today, and I am glad that there is some measure of continuity in the evolvement of our treatment approach.

The following notes are based on the practical experience of the Mulberry Bush School. That such experience should be possible is due to the work of the pioneers in this field; above all, it is due to the work of August Aichhorn, who, having succeeded in modifying public opinion, was able to pursue unorthodox methods long enough to achieve success. He left 'wayward youth' a heritage, namely, the right to expect understanding and help from society in place of condemnation and punishment. We cannot copy him or those pioneers who subsequently worked in this field. However, their individual successes have influenced the opinions of responsible people sufficiently to support new workers like ourselves, who are now able to experiment, with the encouragement and approval of society so that it has been possible for us to permit the damage and await the restitution described in this paper.

Considering first of all the question of attitudes arising in a school like ours in response to aggressive behaviour involving damage, we believe that a tolerant attitude towards all kinds of attack on *things* is necessary while the child is making a 'safe' positive relationship with an adult, thus leaving him free to express the hostile aspects of that relationship against inanimate objects and ideas. Most of the children who come to us have transferred their attacks from people to things. It is therefore undesirable for us to produce a situation in which it will be impossible for them to continue to use this mechanism. Before coming to us, they have probably been severely punished for damage to property; such acts of aggression provided for the time being, a safety valve which they will not need to employ when their attitude towards their parents will have been altered considerably. It is of course necessary during this process to keep a strong framework of community life, to enclose the child and keep him safe. Sooner or later, in fact, when a safe adult relationship is really well established, he will gradually express hostility towards this adult. From this point onwards, as the adult becomes the recipient of aggression and the child begins to value himself as an entity, destruction and damage will tend to occur less often. Once this solid foundation is laid, a long arduous struggle follows, culminating in a more moderate and normal relationship which we must then gradually attempt to transfer to the parents.

Of course it is perfectly possible to forestall the stage of damage and destruction; for example, by introducing the child to an environment which is so 'grand' that any attack on things would be intolerable for him, or to a code of behaviour with a series of sanctions and penalties so well established as to be unassailable.

It seems to me, however, that the heart of the matter lies in being prepared to 'allow things to happen' in order to permit other developments to take place. We have seen the sequence of events to which I refer take place again and again; we do not find the amount of damage done intolerable. We believe that the phase of damage is an essential stage in treatment; we do not believe that the same therapeutic results would be achieved were it possible to acquire completely unbreakable equipment of every kind.

There are certain aspects of such attacks on things which seem to me to be of particular interest, especially in terms of the measure of safety which they provide for the child. Many of the children who come to us are punishment-seeking, and, in consequence, self-destructive. Under certain circumstances it would seem that things can be projections of the child himself, and that in attacking things he can displace fantasy destruction of his own person. For example, an orphan who had spent four years in an institution was deeply preoccupied with his clothes. Under no circumstances could he tear them, dirty them, or lose them; he asked to be allowed to take complete charge of his garments, and was appalled by our own rather casual attitude towards these matters and the indifference of the majority of the children. This boy frequently required treatment for major or minor accidents; he was anxious and afraid of hurting himself, but seemed nevertheless to court physical disaster. After a time his attitude began to alter, and he started to tear and dirty his clothes like everyone else. At just this point he ceased to hurt himself, and actually said to me, 'Isn't it funny? I'm not hurting myself and I'm tearing my clothes.' Another child, a little girl, suffered from severe depressions and was a compulsive runaway. There was evidence of a connection between these flights and a passionate wish that her mother would leave her brutal and psychopathic father. It was either the acting-out of a wish, or a piece of sympathetic magic to make her mother give up her suffering role and run away. She was usually found by the river in a bitterly unhappy condition, and we found that she would always throw some garment—a dress, a shoe, a jersey—into the water. Had we not understood her behaviour, the consequences might have been serious.

Certain things may be symbolic to a particular child and singled out for attack because of their underlying significance. Should such objects be inaccessible, we have no opportunity to observe the particular mechanism. It is especially important that we should be able to do so, because it may actually be this very object which will eventually provide a field for restitution. The boy whom we remember as the 'egg child' is an example of this. This particular child smashed eggs, and this aspect of his behaviour symbolized an attitude to a younger brother which had been present for many years; had the larder been locked we might never have been aware of this fact. At a later date the 'egg child' kept hens!

In observing damage done to objects and attacks carried out upon people, I have been struck by the fact that, just as for certain children things may stand for people, so to others people may stand for things. There is, in this connection, a form of unprovoked attack against a person which does not suggest focused aggression but rather damage done to something which might as easily have been a window or a piece of furniture. I would note that this behaviour can also be positive; for example I have watched a very disturbed child actually using a person as so much play material.

It seems to me that it is essential that the severely maladjusted children in the Mulberry Bush School should thus find their own special outlet for aggression, both for their own sake and because, unless we see these symptoms, we cannot have a complete picture of the child's personality, and so cannot know how best we can help him. I am not suggesting for a moment that there should not be adequate provision for legitimate aggressive activities. These are, of course, essential, but they may not present precisely the opportunities needed by the particular child. I also think that we are unlikely to obtain a clear view of the way in which each child makes restitution unless such damaging behaviour is possible in the first place.

I wish now to consider restitution in its various forms. It is our belief that children who do damage strive consciously or unconsciously to make restitution, which may not be made in the form which is expected and recognized by the unwary adult. What response can the child expect? Should he be punished, and, if not, what can we do instead? One of the most frequent questions asked by visitors of all kinds including officials, parents, students and neighbours is 'What do you do about discipline?'

It is generally accepted that punishment in the form of a

deterrent or retribution has no place in a community of maladjusted children. Enforced restitution is, however, often advocated. We consider that there is a wide gap between enforcing
restitution and making available the means for spontaneous restitution. We feel that our response in any situation should be to the
child's state of mind rather than to his overt behaviour. I do not
believe it is always necessary to make a child aware that he has
committed an antisocial act (as is frequently claimed) since, consciously or not, he will usually be aware of this fact. It may be
argued that other children demand fair play in these situations;
that (for example) the boy who has been attacked demands retribution, or the boy who 'jumps the queue' must be punished because
this is what the group has a right to expect. This is not borne out
by our experience with maladjusted children. It is very often the
adult's point of view which determines the outcome of such situations: we find that the child who has been attacked is completely
satisfied by real sympathy on the part of the grown-up, he does
not demand revenge. It is much more often the adult who seeks
retribution rather than restitution; while the adult may claim that
he represents the group's wishes in asking for punishment, I feel
that there are occasions when it will be found that really it is the
group who reflect the adult's needs in such circumstances.

In the normal course of social development the child accepts
frustration provided that he is compensated with love, he meets
demands in exchange for approval, and, in return for modifications made by the parents modifies his way of life to avoid clashes
with the grown-up pattern. This appreciation of fair play seems to
me to be very important and essentially restitutional amidst so
much that is unfair in the child's world. I have seen one boy
compete with another for affection and approval, each gaining his
needs by fair means or foul; the same children subsequently
playing a nursery game with scrupulous fairness, one taking the
lion's share of attention but dividing the cake precisely in half.
This whole question of what is fair, and what we are justified in
permitting to happen here, often arises in the course of discussion
with visitors. I find that it is very difficult to discuss the question
of response both to damage and to other forms of antisocial
behaviour without arousing anxiety and hostility. In discussions
with all kinds of individuals and groups, I have been struck by

the surprisingly ready acceptance of the concept of restitution in place of punishment. It seems important at this point to stress the difference between enforced restitution and that which is made naturally in answer to the child's own needs. It should also be pointed out that there is a contrast between the making of restitution and self-punishment.

It would seem, from the normal behaviour of young children with their mothers, that there is a trend towards restitution from an early age. Little children do seek to make amends to their mothers. There are circumstances in which we can recognize *regaining* rather than merely gaining approval (which may surely have been lost through refusals to meet mother's wishes and demands, with subsequent guilt arising from feelings of hostility towards the object of their love). What is there so different here from the situation in our school for the emotionally immature child? Here again he refuses demands, is conscious of inadequacy, has hostile feelings and guilt thereafter.

The educational field seems to us to offer a wide variety of means by which restitution can be made (there is so much 'making good' to be done in terms of word building, writing patterns or rows of figures); that this aspect is present in school work has been more than confirmed by our experience here. If the attempts of little children at restitution be unrecognized (as when a child pulls a carrot from the earth and puts it straight into his mother's stew), how much less likely are those of older children to be appreciated in their true light? For example, we once had at the Mulberry Bush a boy who adopted the role of a tender and indulgent mother towards a much smaller child; from what we subsequently learnt about him it became clear that he was acting the part of his own mother making restitution towards her rejected child (himself).

'Normal' children can more easily tolerate the frustrations and demands of moderate discipline including such punishments as may be regarded in the light of enforced restitution, since this is in fact a pattern already accepted by them in the course of development (during weaning and habit training, for example). Should, however, their first experiences have been very unsatisfactory, this clear pattern will not have been formed; although so strong is the trend towards restitution that I suspect that there are frequent cases of distorted attempts to make amends which may even be actually antisocial in character and by no means easy to recognize. Restitution may not be the only component of such attempts. As an example I can quote from the case of a boy of whom we heard who was playing with a clothes line when his younger brother was drowned elsewhere. The death of the younger brother was in no way the child's fault, nor was this suggested by the parents, but subsequently there was a startling change in his personality and very aggressive behaviour became apparent (he had hitherto been a very gentle child). Among other episodes there was one in which he tied up a cat with a piece of rope in a way that seemed cruel. It is possible, however, to detect in this incident an element of restitution; a discussion of his problems in the course of treatment revealed that he felt that he could have saved his little brother with a rope.

When attempts are made to enforce restitution on children with a very abnormal history of emotional development, resistance seems natural: the child has been either building up a strong resistance to his own wishes to make restitution, or he has already satisfied these deep wishes by finding some distorted way of making restitution which will not be recognized as such by others, or, indeed, by himself. He will, therefore, be unwilling–and unable–to adopt a new pattern of response, at first. These are the children who frequently find their way to a school for maladjusted children, and it will readily be appreciated that punishment has no place in their treatment. They need opportunities for destructive activity and for making restitution in their own way. The form which both will take depends very much on the child's particular personality and history. We have found that these children behave in an antisocial manner; they damage, break, steal and the like, but so very secretly that both the antisocial acts and the restitutive activities tend to remain unrelated to the individual children involved.

We find it essential to allow ample scope within the framework of the unit for aggressive behaviour, and at the same time to provide opportunities for various forms of restitution from which the particular child can choose. We do not show approval and we do not adopt any attitude which might suggest approval; but we do accept this behaviour as a necessary step in a process leading back to the meeting of demands and prohibitions of normal life. A small girl said to me, 'Whenever I've been pinching a lot from the larder, it's funny the way I want to work the washing machine.' An older boy, having stolen and opened a tin of plums from the larder, proceeded to give some to a five-year-old, providing a bowl and spoon in the orthodox manner. A girl, having stolen some money from my bag, polished all the furniture in my room. In none of these cases did the children consciously relate the atonement to the desire to make restitution, although it became relatively easy to guess what type of aggressive behaviour has taken place merely by reference to the means of restitution chosen by particular children. I cannot see why it should always be necessary for this kind of reaction to be consciously recognized as such either by the grown-ups or by the children concerned.

It is impressive to note how real and effective a hostile wish may seem to the ill-wisher. I have seen children at the Mulberry Bush make actual amends for fantasied damage, among themselves and in everyday situations. The tacit acceptance of such atonement, whether offered by a grown-up or a child, is often surprising and interesting. Parents who come to the Mulberry Bush frequently make restitution to their children, who may give clear indication that they appreciate the nature of the action. For example, a boy said to me, 'Mummy has sent me a big parcel because she hasn't been to see me recently. When she has been to see me she feels a small one is all right.' Children also show themselves to be aware of these needs in their parents, by making suggestions as to the form the restitution should take; suggestions which may give clues to the relationships existing between parent and child. Sometimes the mother's problems seem to put the child in a position to demand appropriate restitution on her part. We knew an adolescent boy who did not receive much care from his mother in babyhood; in his teens he made demands on her exactly comparable to those of infancy–he demanded from her physical care, money, special meals at odd times, indulgence, comfort and consolation for the smallest trifles; she, weighed down by feelings of guilt, was thankful to acquiesce in these demands in the hope of making restitution for the early deprivations.

I feel, therefore, that by punishing–that is to say, enforcing restitution in some specific form on the disturbed child–the adult may not meet the particular child's needs. He has, in fact, particular things he needs to give as well as to receive: by enforcing the specific form, the grown-up may be replacing the process of atonement natural for this particular child by an artificial form. It is not really necessary for the grown-up to know just how the child will make amends, if he can accept the fact that this will inevitably take place sooner or later, in some form or other. Given a favourable environment, most disturbed children will seek means of atonement suitable to their particular personality problems; since 'make the punishment fit the crime' is a well established slogan, we would suggest to teachers and parents this alternative, 'let him who does damage in his own way make good in his own way'.

To sum up, I suggest that punishment not only anticipates but hampers and probably blocks the natural process of restitution, thereby preventing the further process by which the child may direct into constructive channels the hostile feelings which have led to the guilt and the need for making restitution. Restitution seems, therefore, to me to be a mechanism which may be outgrown as the need for it is removed; enforcing it by artificial means is like using aperients in preference to a healthy diet.

We must now consider some varieties of damage which we encounter in the course of work at the Mulberry Bush, together with the types of restitution we have been able to observe.

First of all there are the children who smash windows, bottles and cups. There are two types of smashers; the child who screams in a tantrum 'all right, I'll smash a window' and does so, and the child who smashes quietly and secretly. We had a boy at the Mulberry Bush who smashed a bottle nearly every day in a particular flowerbed. There are the 'scoopers' who scoop holes in plaster; in this group are often to be found the children who cannot make relationships—the 'frozen children'. The true tearers are always girls; they tear their own clothes, sheets, counterpanes and so on: boys may tear, but usually with a practical end in view. Bed-breakers are another class; not all children vent their hostility on their beds, but certain younger boys tear beds, spring from spring, as it were. Destruction of educational material deserves a discussion to itself; the clean, tidy teacher and the dirty, untidy child, the clean, tidy textbook and the dirty, untidy exercise book have obvious connections.

Tearing of paper increases in the summer months, and the attack on walls and glass lessens. Plants may be pulled up, but not the plants which the children grow themselves. Branches are broken off trees, but this kind of destructive behaviour meets with disapproval from most of the children. It is perhaps worth mentioning the case of an enuretic who actually removed the rubber sheet in order to wet the bed. Tables and chairs seem to get broken through sheer hard use, rather than deliberate damage; cutlery may be burnt or buried—our losses in knives are extremely heavy. Pictures pasted on the walls are torn or defaced fairly soon, usually by small children. However, three posters of flowers remained on the walls for a year, and a row of posters depicting cheerful babies marching along, which was pasted on the wall beside the stairs, has never been damaged in any way during the same period.

Books are preserved astonishingly well by the older girls, but seem to fall to pieces in the hands of boys, and are the objects of savage attack by the very young (of both sexes) who tear them up and burn them. Fires lit by adults are put out by groups of younger children; their own fires, however, survive. Tins of fruit may be pierced with penknives, bags of flour are stabbed, and the inside of a loaf of bread may be scooped out. Eggs are smashed, hair-brushes, clothes and shoes are burned on bonfires; door handles are removed and locks are broken.

This all sounds like wholesale destruction, but let us consider the other side of the picture. Not all the damage is done by all the children all the time; certain children do certain damage at certain times. Children who are recovering show great understanding of damaging behaviour of newcomers. The sum total is by no means disastrous, and we see to it that our equipment is either unbreakable or cheap and quickly replaced. What we have of value is kept out of harm's way.

The spontaneous restitutive activities we have observed include the following. Children help with the housework (bed-making, sweeping and so on), they wash up, do laundry, wash floors or paint, distemper walls, paint woodwork, mend holes in plaster, repair beds, light fires, make cups of tea for grown-ups, give parties to other children, comfort and care for small ones and look after animals devotedly. They save up and spend money on parcels to send home to their families, make themselves very clean, decorate rooms, do jobs of all kinds for people from whom they have stolen (refusing to be paid), produce abnormally clean and tidy work in class, do carpentry (children have told me that wood used for carpentry is 'a tree broken up'), make bowls of clay, etc., for presents to mothers, grow flowers and vegetables which they present to the staff, and buy or cook food for grown-ups ('Here's a cake for the gang'). It does not follow that a bed-mender emerges from a bed-breaker; although this is quite likely it is just as probable that he may be an ardent colour-washer. The girl who steals from me may not return the money, but she is quite likely to buy me a bunch of daffodils, and subsequently be able to speak of the theft and speculate as to its cause. These attitudes have proved perfectly acceptable to our domestic staff, who have the understanding which comes from human warmth and satisfactory experiences.

In conclusion, I would like to refer to the attitudes of visitors of all kinds, from parents to students, towards the damage which we allow to take place at the Mulberry Bush. Parents who have had experience of their child's destructive behaviour and have often used many forms of punishment, mostly need and receive reassurance; they can face the fact that 'here it doesn't matter as it would in your own home'. It is essential that we should help to relieve their sense of failure. The fact that 'this is different' is comforting to them; we are not in competition with the child's home; we speak therefore rather ruefully to parents of the damage done, of the mess and untidiness, at the same time stressing the medical care, the good food, and the outdoor country life. We do not suggest that such destructive behaviour should be tolerated at home; on the contrary, we sympathize with the parents' difficulties. It is one thing to discuss the need for tolerance in the matter of wet sheets . . . it is another to wash them. When clothing is wilfully destroyed we replace the garment; when parcels or presents are stolen, we buy others. When visitors other than parents have to be considered, our comments and explanations depend on the nature of the guest. The truth is really invaluable; for example, when an official asked, 'Why don't you lock your larder?' it was possible to say 'Because then the children couldn't steal food'. It is one thing to note a broken window, but a different matter to learn that Tommy who broke it has an abnormal EEG. We can point proudly to a missing brick at the top of a chimney and say, 'Ah, yes, that was Georgie in his early days, when he started going up rather than out', especially as we can talk of the Georgie of today who comes to visit us during his school holidays, and was described to us by his headmaster as 'such a nice boy'. Some of the most interesting comments we hear are rationalizations made by visitors who are unwillingly attracted to something utterly strange and upside down. A Chairman of an Education Committee remarked: 'I know what it is that I like about that place, it's exactly like a public school.'

The length of the damage-making phase varies considerably in different cases, but it seems reasonably short. As children recover, and their feelings of guilt are relieved, they have less need to make exaggerated gestures of restitution; they help in quite a different way. It is difficult to define this difference, but one is aware that there is no longer an inner compulsion, they tend to ask for a job with pay and do it reasonably well but without desperate zeal. They have passed their *Sturm und Drang* period, and this is apparent in their attitude towards people as well as to things; once a charming delinquent boy, who had a history of a long series of unsuccessful foster homes, said to me (at this point in his progress): 'I've got a new name for you, I'm going to call you Mrs Grumps because you don't have to be wonderful now.' It is the necessity for this weaning stage which indicates how essential it is to have mature workers who can rejoice when they find themselves to be superfluous.

SUMMARY

There are various types of restitution. Firstly, the enforced restitution which is punishment; secondly, the restitution for which means can be made available; thirdly, the fantasy restitution which is carried out by the child in so distorted a way as to be unrecognizable; fourthly, the spontaneous restitution which the child will tend to make according to his own needs. We feel that a school such as ours must be able: (*a*) to make restitution available in various forms, (*b*) to recognize fantasy restitution as a step towards reality restitution, (*c*) to permit aggressive and destructive behaviour under controlled conditions, in order to make possible the return to restitutional trends, with the consequent uncovering of basic feelings of hostility released by making restitution and relief of guilt feelings.

2
Residential treatment
of 'frozen' children, 1958

This paper was built up from a short communication read in 1956 to the British Association of Scientists. I remember my horror and amusement when I found comments on the 'frozen children' in a daily newspaper, which described them as 'leading a Jekyll and Hyde existence'.

In fact, the realizations in this paper proved of very great importance, since the dawning understanding of one category of unintegrated children helped us to recognize others. It was at this point that I met the Winnicotts: I had a discussion with both of them about 'frozen' children, when they confirmed and clarified much that I was as yet only seeing 'through a glass darkly'.

This paper was also published in the British Journal of Delinquency. *I think my main object—in the first place, at all events—was to insist that people should realize what it was like to live and work with such children.*

What follows is based on my findings over the years at the Mulberry Bush School. Various factors have emerged in the attempt to evolve treatment techniques in a residential setting, to help what I would like to call 'frozen' children towards emotional development. These factors have caused me to relate these phenomena to a specific type of disaster experienced at the very beginning of extra-uterine life. Treatment based on my conclusions has been sufficiently successful for it to seem worthwhile discussing its implications.

THEORETICAL APPROACHES

Freud (1926) speaks of the baby's earliest existence in the following terms:

> For just as the mother originally satisfied all the needs of the foetus through her own body, so now, after its birth, she con-

tinues to do so, though partly through other means. There is much more continuity between intra-uterine life and earliest infancy than the impressive caesura of the act of birth allows us to believe.

We believe perhaps too easily that a baby is born because it is no longer *in utero*; no doubt some babies are, as it were, more 'born' than others: but the baby seems to have a second 'intra-uterine' life, the length of which will depend on the nature of the particular unity established as a mother–child entity. Barbara Low uses the term 'nirvana principle', which was accepted by Freud and which sprang from Fechner's concept of a tendency to return to the inorganic. Freud suggests (1926) that the 'nirvana principle' is therefore enlisted in the service of the 'death instinct'. In 1922 Freud wrote: 'The tension then aroused in the previously in-animate matter strove to attain an equilibrium; the first instinct was present, and that to return to lifelessness.' I wish to substitute for 'lifelessness' the word 'selflessness'. I suggest that if a tendency to stability is not regarded as a trend towards a return to the inorganic (lifelessness) but towards selflessness, the whole concept becomes quite acceptable. There is in this case no further need to visualize the child striving to return to the womb; his goal being, in fact, nothing more distant than his mother's arms. I would like to describe this very early period of emotional development as a tactile phase, really pre-oral.

We believe that in the temporary absence of the mother the baby hallucinates her presence, and it seems unlikely that, unless disaster befalls, the baby feels in any way separate from its mother; this would only arise if the baby had to hallucinate for longer than the hallucination could be held (rather like the fading out of hypnagogic imagery). Providing that the concept of the unity can be accepted, we must then consider the transition from the tactile to the oral phase. I suppose that the unity exists during the first weeks of life, and that in normal development there is a gradual withdrawal from it which is so slow and gradual as to pass un-noticed; but made *by the child* with support from the mother, until the emergence of 'me-ness' (Hartmann, 1954 and others). In the case of normal development, it seems unlikely that either mother, baby, or external observer need ever be aware of a state where the baby is neither part of the mother nor a separate entity establishing a dependent object relationship towards her. The whole problem is tackled so gradually that there need never be what a 'frozen' child in the process of recovery once described to me as 'a great gulf'.

Freud has given detailed descriptions of what he calls 'primary narcissism'. He has, however (as far as I know), only made a couple of references to the concept of 'primary masochism'. For example, he writes (1922): 'The exposition I then gave of masochism needs correction in one respect as being too exclusive; masochism may also be what I was there concerned to deny, primary.' And elsewhere (1926) he writes:

> After the chief part of it [the death instinct] has been directed outwards towards objects, there remains as a residuum within the organism the true erotogenic masochism, which on the one hand becomes a component of the libido and on the other still has the subject itself for an object. So that this masochism would be a witness and a survival of that phase of development in which the amalgamation, so important for life afterwards, of death instinct and Eros took place. . . . It then provides that secondary masochism which supplements *the original one*.

Freud links primary masochism with the death instinct, and I am sure that this is absolutely correct, although as he points out, in the course of development primary masochism is not easily to be observed (in contrast to narcissism). I suggest that during the unity the mother's narcissism includes the baby and is so great that it far outweighs any self-destructive tendency; which in any case would not be significantly present in the normal mother (having been dealt with long ago); the baby, as we know, would revive the mother's earlier narcissism, causing her to over-estimate her child. The baby's reservoir of primary narcissism is therefore constantly replenished by its mother from her own store, and the existence of the other reservoir—that is to say, primary masochism—need never become apparent because the narcissistic reservoir does not, as it were, drop its level sufficiently for such an inflow, because of the functioning of the unity.

It is important to stress that the mother's share of the unity is a much more sophisticated version; it is not usually a matter of life and death as it is for the baby who has no other life but that which he shares with her. The withdrawal of either the mother or the baby is felt as an actual loss of self by the other during the period of unity. We know a considerable amount about the mother's experience of a unity. She also is merged; she lives for her child–that is to say, for herself. We know how much her baby seems a part of her; we know how tragically she may react to even his temporary loss as a loss of herself, part of her entity. By the time the unity is finally dissolved and the early object relationship is established, the self-destructive primary masochism of the baby will be projected on to the mother and the outside world; in other words, aggression against self is projected outwards. Some of this aggression will be experienced as direct aggression, some will return against the self as secondary masochism.

I believe that in the so-called 'affectionless' child, whom I prefer to describe as 'frozen' ('affectionless' sounds final, but a thaw can follow a frost), we see the tragic outcome of a disrupted unity, where the baby has been separated from its mother for any one of many causes. We know that in such a case disaster is not inevitable; that another person able to form part of a unity can re-establish this with the baby before it is too late, or better still (as in the case of hospitalization, for example) the mother may be able to re-establish it herself. The disruption of the unity may arise from reality external causes, or it may spring from the personality difficulties of the mother herself, who may be unable to sustain the unity. Our sources of information concerning the other part of a disrupted unity–the baby–must be tapped of necessity in retrospect in the behaviour patterns which are the devices for survival used by the doomed baby, and still used with practically no modification or development by the seven-year-old 'frozen' child.

Every baby, left by himself, will find pleasure and comfort in his own body. I assume that he discovers pain in himself at about the same time or a little later (the finger in his eye, the scratched cheek, and the pulled hair, for example). In normal circumstances, since his mother is part of himself, there is little difference between pleasure in himself or in her. Pain, also, he must associate with her as part of himself, so that when he hurts himself, he hurts the whole unity. However, the balance, as we have already said, is sharply tilted in favour of the pleasure side of the scales. The pain the mother is most likely to cause is negative, in the form of absence; should this be prolonged beyond the scope of self-comfort available to the baby he attacks himself and his immediate environment as *the only part of the unity still available*. Should her absence continue he is thrown back for all pleasure-pain experience on *his limited part of the unity*. This is the secondary role of his body, which, though complete in itself, is only partial in terms of mother–child unity. The resulting situation is one in which self-pleasure and self-pain are more evenly balanced; the desperate dread of self-destruction and frantic hope of self-preservation being the deciding factors in the subsequent history of such a child.

The baby within the safety of the mother–baby unity of the first months of extra-uterine life can, I believe, in the normal course of development experience sorrow, pain, rage and fear; the unity can support these experiences. However, there may be no need for the baby to take the appalling impact of despair, agony, frenzy and panic. The first group of experiences I would like to call 'inner circle', the second group 'outer circle'. I do not believe that in normal circumstances the 'outer circle' group can break through the unity, except for an instant; there are no lasting gaps in the unity of mother–child which acts as Freud's 'barrier against stimuli'. There are, of course, comparable groups on the pleasure side; for example, contentment is 'inner circle', ecstasy is 'outer circle'. Should there, however, be circumstances of either an external reality or of an internal psychic nature to disrupt the unity, then the 'outer circle' can and does break through, and the impact must be sustained. This is what I mean when I speak of a broken unity. Should such a baby develop into a 'frozen' child, I have found that he is unable to be afraid – he panics; he is unable to be sad – he is in despair. I have been with children who are consciously feeling sad or afraid for the first time in their lives, and who need much reassurance in what is to them a new experience. The 'outer circle' experiences have, till their recovery, been of infinite duration while experienced.

A baby who is prematurely self-reliant for all emotional experience does not lose the urge to merge back into the original unity. He does not therefore become a personality within boundaries, as a normal child will do; who comes in the course of maturation gradually to love the mother as a person separate from himself. The child whom we are considering does not make relationships, he does something very much more primitive; he extends and withdraws himself so as to include people whom he uses to provide him with pleasure. He also uses them to ward off pain, by inflicting pain on them, as part of himself, rather than on his very self. Should the person whom he has thus enclosed fail to provide pleasure, he will immediately withdraw; as in the old nursery rhyme, he cries 'This is none of I'. Withdrawals are often mistakenly regarded as breakdowns of relationships, but there has never been a relationship, in the ordinary sense. The behaviour of such children is often described as regressive, when in fact there has been no advance from which to regress.

CLINICAL OBSERVATIONS

A typical 'frozen' child in a therapeutic institution presents a curiously contradictory picture. He has charm—that kind of charm which causes people to say 'I don't know what it is about him. . . .' He is apparently extremely friendly, and seems to make good contacts very quickly. He is neither shy nor anxious in an interview, and in his everyday existence he is usually healthy, clean, tidy and orderly. He is frequently generous and kind to younger children, especially one particular child, whom he protects against all attacks. In astonishing contrast he may become suddenly savagely hostile, especially towards a grown-up with whom he has been friendly. He will fly into sudden panic rages for no apparent reason, in which he smashes and destroys anything in his vicinity (I have known it to be necessary for three adults to control a 'frozen' child in one of these states of frenzy). He is a disturbing element in class—a storm centre—and frequently has acute learning difficulties. Sometimes he seems to build a high wall between himself and other people which is impossible to scale or break through. He steals, lies and destroys relentlessly and without the slightest indication of remorse. It is common to hear workers remark: 'It's impossible to believe it is the same child.' He may manage during one of these periods to continue to show kindness and protection to a particular younger child, but equally he may be cruel to him (in this connection, he is always either cruel or wildly over-indulgent to animals which appear afraid of him). It is repeatedly reported that he is improving and hopes are raised; it is claimed that he is making a relationship at last, but each time disaster follows, until finally he becomes intolerable to his environment. The longer the period of supposed improvement, the more drastic is the breakdown; experience teaches one to think in terms of lull and storm, rather than maturation and regression or recovery and deterioration.

There is another side to the picture which is equally disquieting. The 'frozen' child is, of necessity, delinquent; he may easily become a 'delinquent hero' who gives permission to the other members of the group to break in, steal or destroy. His own lack of remorse, the fact that he can do these things without emotional discomfort, has the most disastrous effect upon all but the most integrated group. In general, the fact that he usually has a current façade relationship has a disrupting influence on an unwary treatment team. (It is very trying to hear the constant comment 'But he is never like that with me'–which in fact only means that his negligible frustration threshold has not yet been reached, the first 'No' has yet to be said!) There often seems to be a conspiracy between child and adult in which the adult is as willing as the child to be unaware of the doppelganger–this monster which suddenly appears instead of the charming child, and which vanishes as suddenly.

This is the picture they present–at seven years, or twelve or sixteen years; there need be no change of pattern, although at seven years the techniques for living this way of life are more apparent than they are at sixteen years, because they are less skilled. Evidence must be looked for in acting out within the environment. There is very seldom any internalized fantasy material available.

Observing this kind of child's behaviour one asks oneself how he can contrive to be utterly without remorse or scruples: how can he live in this state of high tension? We know that he cannot risk being left short of satisfaction for an instant, because the moment that the level of his pleasure drops, pain will flow in. Having withdrawn from frustration he must therefore use any means in his power to maintain the pleasure level, since postponement of satisfaction cannot be risked. It follows naturally that such means will inevitably tend to be delinquent. If, however, the larder door should be locked, grown-ups' pockets empty, or windows securely latched, then crisis will follow, and the second type of merger will take place; in the effort to keep himself from self-destruction he will attempt to destroy his environment, which is felt to be an extension of himself.

Supposing that, as is usually the case, delinquent means are available, how (moral scruples apart) does he ignore inevitable consequences?–there are bound to be disciplinary measures, disapproval and exclusion from the group. The 'frozen' child leads a highly organized and disciplined life, but the organization and the discipline are pathological. There are certain modifications which he has made, and it is precisely these which made it possible for him to maintain some sort of equilibrium.

In the first place, he has achieved what Fritz Redl (1951) terms 'reality blindness'. He does not merely deny that he has done some delinquent or aggressive act, he does not himself know that he has done it. He cannot afford to be aware of any steps he takes to obtain satisfaction; for him there is no gap between instinctual need and the satisfaction of that need. Perhaps it would be more correct to describe this in a more active way as 'selective perception' rather than 'reality blindness'. One recovering child told me: 'I could look at a speck on the wall and not see anything else in the room, and I could always do this with everything.'

Secondly, he has no concept of time. There can be no past to regret, and no future to consider; he lives in the present. He has another safety valve which I have come to think of as 'the reality annexe'. This is represented by an adult, usually on the fringe of the child's environment, whom he uses in a very special way. He uses all his charm on this person, but makes no demands and carries out no reality testing. Frustration never has to be tolerated, because he asks for nothing; instead he satisfies his wishes by delinquent means within his environment, leaving the figure in the reality annexe intact. This provides him with a person who can remain perfect, so that when he is forced to withdraw from one of his extensions by the threat of frustration, he has this almost unreal figure–who is not in the immediate situation–to serve him until he can arrange the next extension. Peter, with a reality annexe B, stole money from us and with it bought presents which he described to us as having been given to him by B. When I showed him what he was doing he broke down in panic, then he was finally reassured and able to tell me that he now realized that he had constantly done this; he gave many examples and explained: 'I can't ask, for fear they say "no", so I don't ask, I just get the things and then they have given them to me.'

The child whom he takes under his wing is an extension of himself; his indulgent attitude is in fact self-indulgence, just as his cruel and punitive treatment of the same child is equally extended-self directed. (We can see here how close the role of protégé lies to that of scapegoat.) His role as delinquent hero secures him material for storm raising, which he does when he is intent on keeping his violence away from himself; on such occasions he is capable of reducing a reasonable group of children to a howling destructive mob. These are all attempts to achieve synthetic unities; he is totally unaware that he uses these techniques – how can he be described as responsible for them?

During the years we have tried to help many of these children. At first we admitted 'frozen' personalities into our group of forty behaviour problems without realizing the implications. We mistook these children for neurotic delinquents, and they caused a great deal of havoc and unrest among staff and children until we gradually became aware of the nature of the problem. We are frequently puzzled as to why certain children are *not* 'frozen'. I know of several cases where, though there was apparently no mother substitute, a little child has been able to become part of a true unity of infinite depth although only of brief duration, which we were actually able through fortunate circumstances to restore. Unfortunately, however, these brief though deep experiences have been interrupted, so that they tend to be a repetition of the original trauma. It is interesting in this connection that Freud expresses his understanding of trauma as being a state of helplessness.

We have slowly evolved techniques for the treatment of 'frozen' children which appear to be successful: we have seen actual changes in their personalities resulting from a particular approach. Indications of conflict have appeared leading to dependence on us, with evidence of deep depression and anxiety (real signs of emotional recovery, since it has long been realized that a delinquent character can only become normal through the experience of a neurosis).

There seem to be two stages of the depressed period. The first is general, and applies to every sphere of the child's existence. He will often become ill, he will be apathetic in every situation and will sit with tears running down his cheeks. He tends to retire to bed; he sits quietly in class, but with no sign of intellectual interest; he altogether presents a tragic picture: this is what we call an 'unfocused depression'. The second part of the depression is different, it is focused on the person with whom the child is now making a primary bond. When this second stage of depression has been reached it is not any longer apparent in every field; the child begins to make educational progress and becomes quite worried and anxious in various aspects of his life. There is, however, the deepest possible attachment to the grown-up of his choice, and in the absence of this person for any length of time the most desperate anxiety is expressed. Disapproval from the special grown-up has become intolerable, and there is evidence of a reaching out towards dependence. Providing that this second stage can be reached, there is little likelihood of reversal, as far as we can see. The earlier stage is by no means so established and the child may revert to the previous delinquent behaviour pattern described.

The second stage of depression and the type of dependence on the grown-up concerned appear to me to have a different significance from that of a transference situation in the usual sense. I suggest that precisely because this is a primary experience there is in fact no transference involved, since there is nothing to transfer. We have, however, had occasion to notice that several of these children who have left us (either to go home, or to another school, or to children's homes) appear to make a transference to a parent figure in the new situation.

With regard to the first stage of depression, I am quite certain that this is a 'state of mourning' for the loss of the unity; the realization that this is something which cannot be regained. It was at this point that a little girl said to me: 'I feel that there is a great gulf which I cannot cross, so now I must go on.' This would represent an experience never really known in normal development, where a baby has ceased to be part of the mother without yet having formed an object relationship with her. The second stage of the depression represents, I think, the establishment of this object relationship. However, it is absolutely essential that the 'frozen' child shall go through the first part of the depression, because at some point or other during this he faces the fact that he has lost the unity for ever, that this cannot be regained. During the later part of treatment (the second stage of depression) when such a child has become an anxious, sad little creature, deeply dependent and infantile, one sees him now and then attempting to use the old mechanisms which now of course no longer function because he has ceased to be 'reality blind'.

An interesting point is that it is remarkable how 'frozen' children who are making a recovery remember most vividly the primary experience through which they have just passed, and they themselves speak of the nature of the mourning and loneliness experienced in the first depression. One child said to me: 'I knew then that I had really been born.' These memories seem to remain extremely vivid, so that several years later children have referred to them, when they have come back to see us. There does not seem to be any amnesia involved, and the memory seems to remain conscious and with very little distortion.

Treatment for this special group is on educational therapeutic lines. At no point is one justified in being merely permissive with a 'frozen' child; one must be controlling, disapproving but not rejecting, approving but not seduced into serving as an extension of the child. At first the behaviour pattern is most carefully observed and reported, until constant repetition of the pattern has made it familiar to the therapist. Next, interruption is introduced; this involves breaking into a behaviour pattern at a critical point in order to make the child aware of what he *has* done, *is* doing, and *plans* to do. A next stage is reached when the first signs of a pattern can be recognized. Each child has a sort of signature tune, which becomes familiar. Interruption now takes place at so early a stage that I think we are justified in speaking of *anticipation*.

James was filthy–he had, I knew, been completely changed just an hour before. However, this was his 'signature tune': he always became dirty before a burst of delinquency. I said quite simply: 'James, go and get clean, you don't have to break in and pinch.' (We knew each other rather well by this time.) He departed to matron and reappeared presently clean and tidy. 'All right', he said, 'have you got a job for me instead?'

Michael played his particular signature tune–a dysrhythmic tapping. I collected him, and pointed out that there was a storm brewing. 'How do you know?' he demanded. I explained, referring to previous occasions, 'You know, I've never noticed,' said Michael. We agreed that he would notice from now on; that the tapping would be a danger signal for him as well. Then we discussed the whole situation, and took measures to avert the storm.

I said to Philip, 'I won't let you hurt George.' I held him and he bit himself–very hard. 'Now see what you've made me do,' he screamed. I had not been quite quick enough on this occasion; I had prevented him hurting George but had not anticipated the inevitable attack on himself.

When interruption or anticipation is used correctly, acute disturbance is felt by the child, and he needs a great deal of support and reassurance. He will do everything in his power to close the gap which has been made in his defences. His response to early interruption is panic and rage, often with actual suicidal threats. If, however, the gap can be kept open by steady interruption and anticipation used in the context of his everyday life, then the next stage may be reached; he returns as it were to the chaos beyond which he has had to isolate himself. Here we meet the first unfocused depression, to which I have made reference, which affects every field of the child's life; during it he re-experiences the loss of the unity and faces the fact that this cannot be restored.

It is at this stage that a kind of bond can be achieved with the therapist; the child becoming utterly babylike, dependent and trusting, completely vulnerable and helpless. It is from this point– and I would assume only from this point–that he can slowly become loving and loved as a complete person (this is the second stage of the depression where it becomes focused on the therapist). One such recovering child said to me one night: 'This bed has an edge like me, but I can put out my hand and hold yours!' This same little boy called kisses 'edges'. 'Give us an "edge"' he would demand, 'I like "edges". They show where I stop and you start.'

I should like to add one example of a particular aspect of the problem which I have described, namely, unawareness of inconvenient reality, and of the measures taken to change this perilous technique for living which is employed of necessity by 'frozen' children.

John (who was nine years old, of average intelligence) had a history of early separation from his mother: there was now the usual picture of a child unable to make relationships, with a severely delinquent behaviour pattern aided by reality blindness, and a highly developed speed of movement (a sort of sleight of person!).

One night, just as he was leaving the bathroom, he threw a clean towel into the bath–which was full. The worker in the bathroom at the time had, by chance, seen this, and called him back to retrieve the towel. John of course did not pay any attention and proceeded singing on his way, after a casual shout of 'No, I didn't'. By now he knew nothing about the towel in the bath. It so happened that I was at the top of the stairs, so taking his hand I said: 'Come on, John, we'll go back together and you can take the towel out of the bath–it's quite safe to know you've done it.' John, usually very cool and tough, became pale, trembled and screamed terrified obscenities at me. I carried him back to the bathroom kicking and shrieking. I assured him again that he really had put the towel in the bath. He continued to scream, and screwed up his eyes. I stayed with him, holding him solidly, re-affirming the facts, and reassuring him; till at last, dreadfully afraid and trembling, he took the towel out of the water. Even now he turned his face away so as to avoid seeing what he was doing, then quite suddenly he gave a great shuddering sigh, wrung out the towel and hung it on the side of the bath. After which he turned to me with a transfigured and radiant face and ran into my arms. I carried him upstairs, tucked him up in bed and he sank almost at once into a deep sleep, still holding my hand.

On another occasion John, who had failed to break into the larder, threw a stone at another child, and flitted round the corner of the house. Having comforted the victim of the attack I picked up the stone and followed John. I held out the stone to him saying, 'This is the stone you threw at Peter.' He stood stock still, staring at the stone, then with great hesitation took it from me and turned it over gingerly in his hand. Finally he said, 'I'm able to hold it, aren't I?'

A child came in sobbing. While I was soothing him, John

appeared at the window. 'It was me what done it,' he said, 'an accident. I'm sorry.' He spoke very quietly and softly, as though afraid to overhear himself.

This child, in becoming instantly unaware of having thrown the towel into the bath, was using the reality blindness which had become so much part of him that he unconsciously employed this defence in every aspect of his life. The therapist, by bringing the defence to a conscious level, made a gap, which produced panic which the therapist then relieved by offering steady support and help to face reality. Constant and consistent repetition of such interruption, and protection, brought John to a point at which he could hold the stone without panic. Finally, we see him at a stage at which he can allow himself to be aware of his motions, although he now rationalizes (he said it was an accident). In the meantime, he has changed from a bright hard young tough—a 'wild one' in the making—to an anxious little boy; stormy, difficult, but deeply attached to a teacher, whose approval he values and whose disapproval causes him pain.

In conclusion, it is my opinion that the psychopath leads a continuation of the desperate existence precariously maintained by the 'frozen' child.

3
Communication as a technique in treating disturbed children, 1959

This is the only paper in the collection of which it can be said that I wrote it for my own pleasure. I was on holiday with the family in North Wales: I lay in bed, or on the sand, or in the heather, and thought about symbolic communication as a therapeutic technique. The actual writing of the paper was done just before our return home, where I found an invitation from the Howard League for Penal Reform to address a course for prison officers in Oxford. I decided to make use of the paper on communication on this occasion: I could see that the subject and presentation could be inappropriate, but I felt more and more that it could be important to talk about what I felt and experienced in the course of my work. This particular audience could not have been more sensitive and articulate: I was glad that I had used this paper which was concerned with inner reality.

> The man in the wilderness said to me,
> 'How many strawberries grow in the sea?'
> I answered him as I thought good,
> 'As many red herrings as grow in the wood.'

This old jingle is an example of communication, in the sense in which I intend to use the word: perhaps content communication would be a more exact description, since it is with the deeper content, rather than with the actual words, that both the communication and the counter-communication are concerned. Thus, although we have no idea what the man in the wilderness was referring to when he asked 'How many strawberries grow in the sea?', and despite the fact that the reply 'As many red herrings as grow in the wood' leaves us equally in the dark, we know that the reply was appropriate and adequate.

I want to discuss communication, using the word in a rather

special sense, as an exact term describing a technique which is of use in therapeutic work with deeply disturbed children, and which I wish to distinguish from interpretation. Interpretation implies a translation of the unconscious content of speech or action into a conscious form available for consideration by the patient and the therapist. As Fenichel says (1945):

> This procedure of deducting what the patient actually means and telling it to him is called interpretation. Since interpretation means helping something unconscious to become conscious by naming it at the moment it is striving to break through, effective interpretation can be given only at one specific point, namely, where the patient's immediate interest is momentarily centred.

Communication does not necessarily involve such translation. The therapist must himself be aware of the interpretation, but–almost simultaneously–he must respond to the communication with regard to its deeper meaning, but in the terms presented to him. Furthermore, the therapist must pick up the emotional content, the 'affect' of the child's communication, and must reply to it with 'affect'–that is to say, without the exchange at any point losing its emotional life. Stereotyped intellectualized responses from grown-ups leave these children in a desert, however 'correct' such responses may be from a theoretical standpoint. I am reminded of the verse about the man who died defending his right of way, which ends:

> He was right, quite right, as he marched along,
> But he's just as dead as though he'd been wrong!

I shall be discussing work which I personally have done with disturbed children; the technique I shall be describing is in use by other members of the team at the Mulberry Bush, and probably by workers elsewhere. I will start at once with a practical example, because this will make the concept clearer.

Little Anne wept when her mother left her at the end of a fairly successful visit. I tried to comfort her, and to find out what was causing such intense distress which was clearly focused on some particular aspect, and much more acute than the grief she usually felt at such times. At last, through her sobs, she exclaimed, 'Mummy only gives me half-a-crown when she comes to see me!'

Half-a-crown was, I knew, a great deal of money to this child; I asked tentatively, 'Wasn't half-a-crown enough, Anne?' She turned on me in a frenzy of despair, crying 'Of course it's not enough, you *know* it's not enough!' I thought of the actual word 'half-a-crown' and was able to pick up the communication she was trying to make, so I replied, 'You need a whole crown?' Anne shrieked 'Of *course* I do!', pummelling me with her fists. I could now answer, 'But you did have a whole crown–long ago, but you really had it.' Suddenly there was a great calm and a shuddering sigh, and Anne said, in her slight, high voice, 'Why can't I remember when I had the whole crown?'

I assured her that though she could not remember her whole crown she had indeed possessed it; furthermore, it was because her crown had been broken rather than outgrown that she felt its loss so bitterly. I also stressed that, broken though it had been, none of it had been given away–that every baby makes with its mother the crown that particular baby needs, and that the mother crowns each baby with the crown they two have made together. Anne nodded gravely, and asked, 'Can we make a crown like I used to wear?' We made one out of gold paper–a very small crown–and Anne, holding it, said quietly, 'Now I know I had one.'

The point I wish to make clear is the fact that this is a very special means of communication between a grown-up and a child, where the child need not be actually aware of the latent in order to make use of the manifest material. It is rather as though one were in a position to accompany and support a dreamer through a dream.

I am sure that mothers use this communication technique with their small children, and that a mother does not need to be aware of what she is doing. Her intuition and her love give her this very special right-of-way through unconscious fields, and this is taken for granted by her child. Each spontaneous communication between mother and child, is, I conjecture, just one part of the adaptation of the total environment which the mother makes for her child; in the very beginning providing a perfect adaptation and gradually failing in adaptation as the baby becomes a separate person (as Winnicott has suggested, 1958, p. 238). The mother continues in some fields to make such adaptation after babyhood, and verbal communication can provide a means for this. Mothers often make apparently irrelevant responses to their little children's statements or questions, which are, however, clearly perfectly correct from the child's point of view. However, this area of communication is lost fairly early, nor is it any longer necessary; the child has, as it were, acquired his own latch-key to himself—to that inner world, the boundaries of which are so closely guarded by the normal person.

Other people besides mothers use the technique now and then in an intuitive way. People who work with children and who tend to be described as 'very good with children' pick up and respond to communications without noticing that they have done something special. Workers in my own particular field—the residential treatment of disturbed children—also use this method, but because they tend to work in an intuitive way they usually find it difficult to answer the question which is so often asked: 'Just what do you do?'

The danger of such intuitive communication, be it maternal or otherwise, lies in the fact that it is only too easy for a disturbed mother or worker to pick up the latent content of a child's communication and respond to it in terms of the adult's own inner world, so that a no-man's-land may be created, shared by mother and child or worker and child. This is liable to be at a great cost to the child, because he may become the one who has to produce the correct responses; lacking resources and a clear boundary to his inner world, he may be exploited by mother or worker, who will be unaware of the harm being done. Intuition informed is an essential tool: intuition uninformed can be a dangerous weapon.

The therapist working in a residential treatment setting is in many ways comparable to a mother with her baby, and faces many of the same problems. The most important of these problems is that of survival: it is a matter for wonder that mothers *do* survive, that their babies do not in fact 'gobble them all up', and that a mother can go on apparently giving away the whole of herself and yet preserving the whole of herself for the next ruthless onslaught. The point is, I feel, that the mother does not in fact give herself away, but the baby's own 'herself', which her child has created with her following the earliest phase when mother and baby are one.

The therapist also has to give all and yet survive complete, and not only for one particular child but for several other children each just as particular. This complete survival is not always achieved, and therapists can break down under the strain–they lose themselves. It is obviously essential that the therapist should be well aware of what he is doing; he must neither be lost in the child's inner world, nor allow the child to slip over the threshold into his own. This implies that the therapist has gained knowledge of his own inner world: without such knowledge there cannot be informed intuition. However much the therapist knows about himself, there will still be some children whose communications he can pick up more easily because they are, as it were, in his own language: but the more he knows about himself and the more experience he gains, the greater will be the variety of the communications which he will be able to pick up from children whom he can understand and love–and even hate now and then–without danger to himself or to the children.

Another problem which the therapist must face is that the child is not in fact a baby; the actual holding in the arms, the feeding and the wrapping must all be limited in their overt forms. The therapist is faced with the need to provide an apparently tough, sophisticated ten-year-old delinquent with an environment approximating to that which failed him when he was a few months old; communication is one technique for achieving this aim. The child with whom such contact is established feels–correctly–that this is his own absolutely personal and deep connection with his therapist: it even feels for him at some points that he and his therapist are contained within the field of their communication. By preserving his own identity, and by holding separate 'lifelines' for each of his contacts, the therapist can adapt to the inner needs of each child in this deep though limited way, which is so much more a matter of quality than of quantity.

Michael went through a long intensive period with me during which we sorted out the tangled skeins of his devastating memories and 'forgettings'. Later on, he came to see me at intervals; he would come into my room, smile at me, and demand 'Ask me to do sums!' There was, however, only one sum which I should ask for–'What do one and one make?' To this he would reply every time, with tenderness and sadness, 'They make one.'

This was the all important sum of his mother and himself as a little baby.

I have said very explicitly 'the therapist in residential treatment', and I do not suppose that this technique would be generally applicable in other spheres of therapeutic work; apart from anything else the communication is always made and received *in context* rather than in retrospect. It is at that instant in time and space that the response must be made and the adaptation provided. Postponement is as impossible for such a child as it is for a baby. The therapist is dealing with *this* happening *now*, not with *that* happening *then*, however closely one may in fact relate to the other.

Thus, had I told Anne that in talking about the half-crown she was referring to the breakdown of the bond between herself and her mother (which took place when Anne was in hospital, in most traumatic circumstances) I would have achieved nothing except to provide her with information which she already possessed. She was well aware of her frantic jealousy of her younger brother, at a certain level, but the half of the crown which she feared that her mother had given to him was another matter. Again, she knew that she had experienced an early security (which was in fact what had saved her from total disaster) but she had not realized that each baby and mother create something unique for themselves. What we achieved together was an understanding of these matters in Anne's own language; so that what had been, as it were, 'outside' general knowledge became 'inside' and special, and in a form in which it could be preserved. I also think that the communication took place below the level of her defences, which made it practical for Anne to know and yet not to know what had happened to her.

I must at this point mention something which I have come to recognize as a fairly constant phenomenon but which I do not really understand, namely, the significant comment or response. How *does* the therapist recognize this among all the minute-to-minute verbal activity? I am sure that there is a particular quality about the way in which significant phrases are said–perhaps because of the very heavy load of emotion which they carry. In the case of Anne and her crown this was of course very obvious; in most cases, however, the communication is by no means so easily noted, and could easily be missed—as, alas, I am sure these cries for help *are* missed or misunderstood by all of us. There is, nevertheless, comfort in the fact that once the child wishes and needs to communicate something he will continue to attempt to establish contact; once this is established the child will expect the therapist to respond suitably and will be impatient and critical if one loses the thread of his pattern. This tends to ensure continuity where this is required; there may be a series of communications on a theme, but again there may be an instant of communication that is tremendously important though isolated.

A group of small disturbed children made little nests from straw and twigs, which they brought to me to ask for eggs to put in the nest. I divided a large bar of chocolate into small squares, and asked the first child 'How many eggs for your nest?' 'Four', he replied (no doubt for excellent reasons). The second boy replied 'Five'. The third, however, who was in fact extremely greedy, replied 'One'. The chocolate was much more an egg for him than a piece of chocolate, and he wanted to be the only egg to be laid in the nest! This was very evident from the way he tenderly tucked the piece of chocolate into the nest, and it was still there long after the other 'eggs' had been eaten. It would have been a serious mistake for me to have pressed him to have more chocolate, and to have commented would have been unnecessary intrusion.

I assumed at one time that communication could only be used where the therapist already had a great deal of knowledge about the child, as I possessed in Anne's case. Later, however, whilst carrying out a piece of research, I had a series of single interviews with children about whom I had little or no information. I had many interesting experiences, but one was especially remarkable: a boy of nine brought me a picture of a house perched in the bottom of a ravine. For an hour we talked together about the house, of his chances of finding a guide with whom he could face the dangerous ascent of the far side of the ravine, and of his terrifying descent from this side which he had only made because he knew that behind him lay the vast and limitless desert which he had traversed for eternity. 'And beyond this desert?' I asked. He replied very hesitatingly that there was a warm and wonderful country, but so long ago . . . so far away. . . . We agreed that this golden age could be mourned but never regained. In the meantime there were, it seemed, guides in the house–one in particular. 'When the spring comes we may try the other side, I think there are footholds.' I am sure that he did in fact find the footholds on the other side of the ravine.

Another child told me how cold he often felt; it was clear that this was no ordinary cold of which he spoke, and I had the impression that there had been a time when, like Kay in Hans Andersen's 'Snow Queen', he had been too cold to feel at all. I told him this and said, 'You know, if you were still frozen you would not be able to feel the cold; it is because you are thawing that you feel this great pain. One day, when you have quite thawed, it will be different–at present I'm afraid it must hurt very much.' We talked a little longer and he went away, but I heard a sequel from his own 'special' person in the institution where he lived. Apparently he went at once to find this person, and said with tears of gladness, 'She comforted me. I'm thawing and getting better, that's why it hurts.'

I guess that in cases such as this the child has managed to pick up some mutual kind of wavelength in order to reach the therapist. Clearly, the more skilled and experienced the worker becomes, the more likely he is to be reached and to be able to reach back without anxiety. This initial recognition of a significant communication remains intuitive–a *Fingerspitzengefühl*–the therapist cannot set out to pick up communications, he must wait for them; but he can create a favourable climate in which communication can take place, and be receptive and constant, always with something to give, something to take, and something to keep for himself.

Margaret, aged thirteen, had been a 'frozen' delinquent child, but had 'thawed', so that now there was a fragile little self of which she took great care. She never spoke of this self of which she was now deeply aware, but she talked of a little cat called Gigi in such a way that I was sure that Gigi was being used to house the new-found self.

One day we went together to visit the clinic where she had received valuable treatment at an earlier stage of her life. We had breakfast on the train and Margaret was very poised and grown-up. Presently, however, she said in ordinary and rather businesslike tones, 'Would you please put Gigi in your brief case?' I said 'Of course', and, taking the case down from the rack, put the invisible Gigi in it and replaced the case on the rack. Margaret thanked me, and asked me now and then during the journey whether Gigi was safe. As we crossed London in the underground she told me to keep Gigi safe for her while we were at the clinic. I said I would gladly do this, but that in fact Gigi would by now be safe with Margaret herself–that one day she might even be contained by Margaret. 'Perhaps,' said Margaret, 'but not yet.' In the end she felt secure enough to take Gigi *in* my brief case, and carry her into the clinic.

I have said nothing so far concerning the kind of relationship involved in a communication technique such as I have described. The children with whom we work at the Mulberry Bush are for the most part extremely rudimentary personalities, especially the group which I call 'frozen' and which is made up of real delinquents, the hard core of any treatment group. They have never made a real bond with another human being; they have little or no 'inner world', they use their immediate environment instead; they are in no position to establish communications because they have no inner equipment with which to do so. Nevertheless, it is eventually possible with just this group that communication can be most successfully established, but only following the first stage of treatment during which, far from producing an adaptive environment, it is necessary to render useless all their successful but pathological techniques for living.

The aim of the therapist is to establish the identity of the child, to push him back within the boundaries of himself whenever he attempts to merge with his environment. This is a very difficult and painful process which must be passed through in order to reach the vital point at which the child can feel a deep sorrow and a complete dependence on his therapist. It is at this stage that communications are made most freely; the first often concerns the barrier between inside and outside reality felt by the child as an 'edge' to himself, or the vast space which he feels lies between him and other people, across which he must be prepared to reach the therapist. He refers to isolation and helplessness and to the terrors of infinite time and space. Such a communication was made by the boy who brought me his picture of the house in the ravine; in which he referred, in fact, to the isolation and helplessness which he experienced as a baby prematurely divided from his mother.

As with a very little child, so with our 'unfrozen' delinquent, the barrier between inside and outside himself is very fragile. The existence of the strengthening primary bond between child and therapist provides the necessary channel for establishing contact. As the child's inner world becomes richer and more separate from outside reality it also becomes more hidden and secret, as it would with a small child during normal development.

I have spoken elsewhere of the difference between a primary bond and a transference; here I would only remark that in my view there can be no question of a transference being established with a child who has never had the experience of loving someone else as a separate person. The word transference implies transfer *from*, and such a child has nothing *from which* to transfer. The term primary bond is a description of the first bond that a baby makes with its mother, having emerged from a state of unity with her. It is just such a point that a 'frozen' delinquent must reach, and it is a *progress* rather than a regression which he makes, because he has never really reached integration before; he is having *first* experiences, since it was at the earliest unintegrated stage that his development was interrupted. Once a primary bond is established and communication is achieved, it is important to realize that even this achievement is by no means total recovery. In fact, what we feel we can honestly claim is that we have made it possible for the child to be neurotic, with the hope of ultimate recovery through the ability to make dependent relationships, having reached Klein's depressive position (Klein, 1944) which Winnicott describes as 'the stage of concern' (Winnicott, 1958, p. 206). Ideally, such a child should later have further treatment (when transference and interpretation would come into their own), but at least he cannot easily return to his earlier 'frozen' state, and is unlikely to grow up into a psychopath.

My impression from my own work, and from that of other members of our team, is that the therapist working in terms of a primary bond is not faced by certain difficulties inherent in a transference situation. Firstly, there will be no skilful resistance nor elaborate system of defences (because of the primitive stage of ego development reached by such a child): secondly, there will not be ambivalence in a mature sense, because it has not been reached. Hate in this primary experience is primitive self-hate projected onto the therapist, which, uncomfortable as it certainly is to experience, is infinitely less wearing than the complex love–hate mixture of the more mature personality, if only because it can be seen at once since it is scarcely disguised. Thus the child accuses the loved therapist of being quite ready to let him starve, or be lost for ever, or drown in the river; what he needs at first, rather than interpretation of the mechanism of projection (which may drive him into suicidal behaviour) is reassurance that the therapist will pull him out of the river, feed him, and find him when he is lost. (It is quite likely that the therapist may have in reality to do these things at some point!)

I am clear that the establishment of a primary bond, with all it implies, and the achievement of communication must be accomplished before there can be any change in a delinquent personality. Sometimes we are unable to help the child to do this, despite all our efforts, and the result may be a superficial adaptation but not in any sense a complete recovery.

I have especially discussed 'frozen' children because it is with them that I do most of this sort of work, but the same kind of approach may be suitable for certain types of psychotic episodes. I have also worked with several gifted neurotic children who have appeared to use the same methods of communication, but in fact have done something quite different, usually conscious, and akin perhaps to the poetry of the so-called metaphysical poets. 'As if' is implied if not actually quoted; the child is choosing ways of making the meaning of difficult concepts clear to himself and me. In a case like this the therapist and child may choose to discuss problems within the chosen symbolic framework, but sooner or later direct interpretation will certainly be made by the therapist or by the child.

I have described the more usual ways in which children make communication; the examples given are of necessity rather simple, because the more complex systems would require a lot of explanation. However, brief descriptions of two such complex systems may show how they are evolved by children. One was developed round a simple drawing, the other round the child's own name.

It will be seen from the following brief excerpts how difficult it can be to notice the necessary clues.

James used to come and see me frequently in order to have very superficial, sophisticated conversations and to scribble a certain little picture while he chattered to me about nothing at all. The picture was a drawing of a small boat on a sea; there was nothing special about the boat, which was stereotyped, the drawing never varying in the slightest particular. Nothing that he said while he was drawing gave me a clue, but I continued to feel that I was failing to collect something of vital importance every time he came to see me. I do not remember what eventually made visible the key which he put into my hand each time he came but one day I asked him, 'Where are you standing?'

James: 'Down there' (pointing to some air below the picture).

Myself (feeling my way cautiously): 'What is beneath your feet?'

James: 'Stone–a quay is always made of stone.'

Myself: 'Is the boat always just there?'

James: 'As far as I know it is–I think it is anchored there, out in the bay.'

He went on to tell me more about the town and the people who lived in it–a whole complicated inner world, which was very important and very hidden, except for *the view he could see from the quay!* In the town and its environments James preserved his emotional experiences. As I came to know the houses and the people, so also I came to know something about his early life. It will be noticed that James had a more complex and developed personality, able to preserve memories in the form of symbols. The only *communication* made was contained in the drawing of the boat; the fantasy of the town and the harbour already existed, and could be interpreted once reached; the communication was therefore a stepping-stone.

The other small boy was called Anthony Rock. One day he was talking about the meaning of names in such a way that I asked him what his own surname meant to him. He replied 'The edge of a rock', and spoke of the dangers of falling off the rock into the sea below. Later we reached a point where we could consider fine days when he could climb down the rock safely and sail across the sea (he had never thought of the rock as something to be climbed up or down, only as something over which he could fall to his death). He pointed out that if he were to set sail we ought to build a lighthouse on the rock, so that he could find his way back. We found a night-light, by great good fortune, made in the form of a lighthouse, which I bought for him, and which became a talisman.

I have tried in this paper to extract one technique, which I have called communication, from the main branch of residential treatment of disturbed children. I must stress the fact that I have only been discussing a cross-section of the total treatment which we at the Mulberry Bush call Context Therapy; I must also stress that communication—however exact and well-established—would never be adequate by itself, and must be combined with very special and skilled management in every sphere of the child's life.

SUMMARY

The word communication is used in a very special sense to describe a technique employed in a certain kind of treatment of deeply disturbed children, in a residential setting.

Communication *with* is distinguished from interpretation *to* a child, because while interpretation brings *latent* content to the surface, communication while concerned with latent content is carried out in terms of *manifest* content.

Such communication can be established between a child and the therapist. It is most likely to appear following the formation of a primary bond.

It is practical for one therapist to maintain several of these lines of communication at the same time; this is therefore an emotionally economic technique. The fact that the therapist can respond to the child at once, in context and with feeling, provides just the kind of adaptation to needs that a very disturbed child needs at a certain stage of treatment. The therapist can continue to maintain such a contact without too much strain, each child having his own highly individual lifeline which he will be inclined to hold very firmly.

Mistakes—inevitable in every kind of treatment—are not disastrous, once contact is established. Before this point there is no communication in the special sense, and after this point the child will correct mistakes.

Mothers and certain gifted people have such means of making contact with the inner world of children; this intuitive skill tends to be lost as the child concerned grows up and inside and outside become more firmly established. The therapist, like the mother, must be able to tolerate the eventual loss of the lifeline when it is no longer needed.

Some children will have a whole system of communication, others may have moments of contact which are just as important.

Story-tellers and dreamers have been making communications since the beginning of history. We are often concerned with the interpretation of these myths or poems, or whatever we choose to call them. Perhaps there are times when we should simply respond to them as communication.

Progress is made from pre-integration to integration. (For example: Jane, who had been a 'frozen' delinquent, read the fairy-tale in which, in order to gain a soul, a fairy must sacrifice her immortality. In recounting this story Jane said: 'You know, this is what happened to me.' Because she now knew of a tomorrow and a yesterday she knew also that she was born and would die—she had lost the 'immortality' of the psychopath who lives entirely in 'today'.)

Interpretation seems to belong to transference and (probably) regression towards disintegration; communication belongs to a primary bond and progress towards first integration.

4

The outsider and the insider in a therapeutic school, 1960

We have always valued the link established with the Tavistock Clinic early in the history of the Mulberry Bush, in terms of referral and psychiatric supervision. During 1958 and 1959, Elizabeth Brown, a tutor psychiatric social worker at the Tavistock, ran a monthly discussion group at the Mulberry Bush. The paper which follows is a description of this project, from my point of view within the school: Miss Brown also wrote a paper on the same subject but from her standpoint as the leader of the group. We both read our papers to a conference of the Association of Psychiatric Social Workers: both papers were published subsequently in 'Ventures in Professional Co-operation'.

I am going to discuss the effect of outsiders on insiders in a therapeutic school. This seems to me to be a very important subject and one which I am anxious to understand more clearly myself, because I think the problems which I shall be discussing apply to the work of anyone who is at any time an outsider crossing the threshold in order to come inside a home, a school, a clinic, or any containing environment concerned with dependent relationships. The problem as I see it, is simply this: that an outsider does not turn into an insider by coming within. In other words, he or she, having crossed the threshold will be an 'outsider inside'. What happens after this point is reached will depend on the factors which I am trying to consider in this paper.

Most of us who are working with people are insiders in terms of our own frame of reference. We usually belong to a group or a team, which is united in the attempt to help other people; sometimes, indeed, to help them to cross thresholds themselves in order gradually to become insiders within a family or a social group. I am trying to present to you (as far as I can bear this) a fairly uncensored account of my own personal feelings during a particular experience as an insider.

TYPES OF ENCOUNTER

There are three types of visitor likely to turn up in a therapeutic school.

1. Those who come in at one door and go out at the other without doing more than establishing a superficial or tangential kind of contact which evokes a counter-contact.
2. Those who come in and establish themselves, making an impact and producing a response.
3. Lastly, there are those who break through, or impinge, producing a reaction.

The terms used above are descriptive words rather than psychological terms, in this context. Response and reaction have acquired various special meanings as technical terms ('conditioned response' for example). Here I am using these words in accordance with some of the meanings attached to them by the dictionary, or by general usage. Thus it is usually accepted that a reaction is more violent, more primitive than a response, whether it is positive or negative.

What I am really saying throughout this paper, is that it can be deeply disturbing to the insiders for outsiders to come inside, but that there are ways of entering which are *not* disturbing.

People working with what I have described as pre-neurotic children are extremely vulnerable, because of the tremendous personal involvement necessary in working with regressions and progressions. At certain points in this kind of work the adult is as undefended in relation to the child as a mother usually is in relation to her baby. It is painful and difficult to discard such defences even for the time being, and can only be relatively safe in a highly protected environment. The mother–baby unity is vulnerable in the same way. This unity is protected (all being well) by a barrier against stimuli provided ideally by the father, or failing him, by other protecting people and by the home milieu itself. The therapist–child involvement must also be protected by a supporting person (whom I find it convenient to call the catalyst), and by the therapeutic milieu. The catalyst is the person who can be used by both the adult and the child, remaining constant and unchanging, and thus facilitating deep changes in the involvement of adult and child.

The danger to both mother–baby unity and therapist–child involvement is impingement, that is to say, a break through the protective barrier which surrounds them. This is a *real* danger to their inner world, and the fear is a *real* fear, and thoroughly justified. I think that in such circumstances we should learn to respect what appears to be a defensive and suspicious attitude, and see that it may be normal in this special context, because of the inner realities of the involvement.

The in-at-one-door-out-at-the-other type of visitor is nothing worse than an irrelevance. The breaker-in, however, is liable to crash through the barrier protecting both the general therapeutic milieu and special involvements within it, producing reaction (panic, rage, despair), and doing severe damage at a deep level, which may be difficult to make good. The visitor who makes an impact may evoke a response (either positive or negative) from those who are involved, but will not damage the involvement itself, which is going on at a deeper level. Miss Brown's work with our team is an example of this, but before discussing it I would like to give examples which we have experienced of contact and breaking-in.

Contact. A teacher from another country came to spend a month with us. This was her first visit to a school for maladjusted children, but she had read a lot about progressive schools and expected the Mulberry Bush to fit within such a frame of reference. On the eve of her departure I was amazed to find that she had been able to see the Bush exactly as she had expected, in spite of her opportunities to observe the children, and discuss and read about our work and aims. She had come, and was going, without anything having happened to her or to us. She had been extremely nice, had caused no disturbance, but neither had she made any impact on us, or we on her. Here, then, was an outsider who had come inside, and nothing had happened.

Impingement. This is often quite unconscious; it is possible for the outsider to enter the group in a way which, at a conscious level, is friendly and positive, although at an unconscious level this is a destructive act, and is experienced as such by the group.

On one such occasion, Mr A, the warden of a hostel for mal-adjusted children, came unexpectedly with two members of his staff to visit a child called Tom. He was welcomed by one of the team, Miss C; she was about to look for Tom when suddenly Mr A exclaimed, 'What happens in there?' and the three outsiders plunged straight into the middle of Miss C's group, leaving her for an instant *outside* her group and separated from it by strangers to both herself and the group. Miss C handled the traumatic situation very well, but of course both she and the group experienced a reaction. Here an outsider came inside, and did harm.

IMPACT: THE DISCUSSION GROUP

We can now settle down midway between contact and impingement, and consider impact and response, in terms of Miss Brown's discussion group.

When she became a director of the school, Miss Brown and I worked on the plan for her to lead a monthly discussion group with the Mulberry Bush team. The team liked the idea very much, and the discussion group became an established and enriching part of life at the Mulberry Bush.

Miss Brown's paper was concerned with the history of her work with this group. Here I shall be thinking about my own personal experience as a member of the group, a supporter to the team, a principal of the school and an insider.

There were certain favourable factors which made it easier for me to be a member of this group than might otherwise have been the case. Miss Brown is a family friend, thus a solid foundation already existed for the work together at the Mulberry Bush. We have always been able to accept the fact that we have different theoretical views, and are not inclined to tread often, or heavily, on each other's emotional toes. Not only was she known person-ally to me, but she had frequently come to the Mulberry Bush; she had become friendly with some of the team, both at the Mul-berry Bush and at refresher courses organized by the Association of Workers for Maladjusted Children. She was, moreover, already aware of the general trend of work at the Mulberry Bush and of our particular set of values, and was identified with our aims. Being a director, she was aware of periods of stress for the school, financial and otherwise, which we could not otherwise have revealed. We have worked with the Tavistock Clinic since the early days of the school; various Tavistock people including Miss Brown herself had given us a great deal of help and advice, so that there was already a strong link between clinic and school.

There were also certain difficulties for me in the situation. I was both the principal of the school and a member of the group. The fact that I was not an authority figure in the school made the situation, for the group and myself, even more complicated than it would have been had I been a principal in the usual sense of the work. Had I remained out of the group, however, this would have made even greater difficulties for all of us, for obvious reasons. The fact that I knew Miss Brown well, had advantages and disadvantages for the group, who knew of course that Miss Brown and I met outside the group situation. I knew a good deal about various members of the team, who naturally needed and received from me (as catalyst) individual therapeutic support from time to time: such knowledge I had no right to impart, but neither could I be unaware of its implications in the group situation. My position was, therefore, complicated because my function in the group was in no way therapeutic, and this could be difficult for any member of the team who might at that particular moment happen to be emotionally dependent upon me. While I was myself a catalyst supporting current involvements in the Mulberry Bush, I was receiving support in my *own* current involvements in the course of work I was doing *outside* the school, from my supervisor (within the school, the particular children with whom I was working had either, as it happened, integrated already or had not reached a stage of involvement with me). Although the theoretical differences of opinion between Miss Brown and myself were not fundamental (and we both tried to avoid arguments about psycho-analytic theory) the group was inevitably aware of these differences from time to time. During this period I was gradually grasping certain ideas, such as those discussed above, and others which I have written about elsewhere, but was not yet ready to discuss them with the group: I felt very hampered by this and often resentful, especially when I very unwisely tried to talk about these partially conceptualized experiences.

Many of the problems which I have outlined arose only occasionally, because of the special quality of the group, determined I think, by facts which I have overlooked.

In the first place, Miss Brown could only come once a month, so that the tensions characteristic of therapeutic groups were less likely to turn up; this was recognized by all concerned to be simply a discussion group. Secondly, discussion took place after supper, when we were all very tired after a long day's work; we found the discussions both refreshing and stimulating, partly because they did not take place in the context of the day's urgent minute-to-minute experience, and consequently provided a change of atmosphere.

In this setting we discussed events and feelings *in retrospect*, and I noticed that none of us talked about involvement and reaction because this was really too painful and disturbing to be evoked out of context (and, indeed, in context all that one can do with reaction is to know one is reacting, and such knowledge would often be denied or rationalized later, because of its intolerable nature). Accordingly, both Miss Brown and the group functioned in terms of impact and response. We left severely alone the Ultima Thule of involvement and the problems of unintegrated experience, and concerned ourselves with the vast area covered by consideration of transference and counter-transference.

Withdrawal of concern was spoken about, although not acknowledged as such, while the experience of involvement and the threat of impingement were not mentioned. This withdrawal of concern is a betrayal of commitment just as traumatic as impingement. I would say that conscious involvement with concern is essential where primary experience is required: involvement, whether conscious or not, without concern is in fact a delinquent type of merger, and dangerous; withdrawal of conscious concern from an involvement is traumatic.

There were of course many children in the school who had reached integration, and for whom considerations of secondary experience were of the utmost importance (by 'secondary' here, I mean post-integration, but still very early experience, such as introjection and projection).

I remember wondering at the time to what extent involvement *could* be discussed in a group. In fact, when staff members come to me for individual support they do not discuss involvement. They are suffering from it; from the pain and shock of reaction to primary unrepressed hate (for example), and the resulting emotional impoverishment. What they need is support and emotional 'first aid'. Adults involved with children can only risk their own inevitable failure in adaptation to needs, if they can be certain of the supporting catalyst in the background, to assure them that this failure is inevitable and not a disastrous letting-down of children in treatment. During this period one member of the team was consciously deeply involved with a child working through a localized regression, and needed constant emotional refuelling, being under tremendous stress. References to this particular child were made by the adult concerned from time to time, both in the discussion group and outside; but only when we were alone could I see clearly the depth of experience for adult and child.

I think that this sort of thing is comparable to watching a mother feeding her baby. One becomes aware of watching an observed mother and baby, and of being outside the 'nursing couple' zone; one is, of course, extremely careful not to break through the barrier which one is as it were already bending by one's presence. It will, however, be perfectly possible to talk with the mother about her baby and herself in this situation. She responds to the impact, and communication occurs at a tolerable level, where there is no question of impingement.

This was exactly what I think Miss Brown did; although, in her respect for the therapeutic situation and the sensitivity of the individual workers, she limited the depth of discussion. This made it possible to talk about a great deal in reasonable emotional comfort, and without the erection of further hampering defences to ward off possible impingement. A group doing work less emotionally loaded than ours would not be living under this particular kind of strain; the members would be neither involved nor reacting, except occasionally, so that for them such a discussion group might prove an outlet for *potential* reactions. (I do not feel it would be too far-fetched to compare our experience with that of the disturbed children in our care, who spend such stormy days that they have remarkably peaceful nights!)

An outsider who was less sensitive, knowledgeable and aware, might have broken into the inner world of an involvement, and it is dreadful to contemplate the damage which could be done by a clinical bulldozer in this sort of field.

There were of course moments when I was disturbed in the group – when I felt threatened as a therapist or as a catalyst supporter, by some turn in the discussion. On one occasion, for example, a theoretical argument took place about the concept of perfect emotional adaptation in a mother–baby unity. This concept was already axiomatic for me, but not yet really accepted by the team; even though some of them were themselves making these adaptations (perfect though localized) in the context of treatment, and were just starting to be aware of the difference between involvement and transference as a result of experience, but had not yet realized it consciously.

I was, thanks to my analysis, quite conscious of my own emotional state in bringing a child through a regression, but nevertheless this did not mean that I could avoid being in such a state, essential as it is to conscious involvement.

It seems absolutely necessary for people who are learning how to work through a regression or progression to have such experience, followed by realization followed by conceptualization, in that order; so that if now and then an idea turns up before, or during the experience, argument about the idea can produce anxiety about the not-yet-realized experience. Thus, I was sometimes presented in this way with a double problem; for myself personally, as a therapist involved in a regression, and also as a catalyst supporting adults and children who were experiencing involvement, but who had not yet reached realization. It was perhaps especially difficult for me at that time because I was deeply involved with a child in a total regression outside the Mulberry Bush, so that I was myself very vulnerable and sensitive in the special way that I have described. Although I did not mention this at the time to anyone it must have affected the group situation. I was indeed conscious of this, but although I was already used to these phenomena of regression I was in too sensitive a state to be able to discuss this sort of thing objectively until the child and I were out of the 'trough' of the regression. Another reason for my silence was that the team depended on the illusion of my reliability for their security in their own involvements. Any discussion at this point about matters too near the bone emotionally for me affected me like an impingement, although of course it was really nothing of the kind.

It was a very real problem for both Miss Brown and myself that she did not know much about the actual therapeutic work which I was doing; nor, at that point, could I explain it to her. There is nothing more hopeless than an endeavour to communicate experiences which have only just been realized. A difficulty here was that of vocabulary, as she herself pointed out I tended to use in special ways terms already in use in other ways, which was of course most unsatisfactory.

Another disturbing occasion for me was just before my own family moved from the school to a house of our own, at the end of the village. This move affected everybody in different ways. For one staff member the fact that we were no longer going to be living in acute discomfort made it difficult to identify with us. For another, only our constant presence in the school made it possible for other people to go away, or be ill, and so on, because concern could be as it were shifted on to our shoulders. Our move pushed back a sudden load of personal responsibility on to each individual member of the team. There was also, of course, our own personal guilt; the feeling that we would be letting down the team, the school and everything else, by taking this step, combined with omnipotent notions that only if we were living in the Mulberry Bush could it in fact survive! The reality was of course very different. The whole subject surfaced in the group, and I felt very much, at the time, that this was something to be faced individually rather than by the group as a whole. Here my own feelings of personal guilt came in very strongly, although I think perhaps I was right in terms of the group.

We were all deeply concerned when Miss Brown had to leave us because of her mother's illness. Although we had only met once a month, her initial relationships with some members of the group had been strengthened and deepened during this period; and new relationships were just beginning to grow with the other members. The fact that this was not a therapeutic group did not, of course, prevent deep emotional experiences taking place within it (Miss Brown, while aware of and responsive to such experience, did not interpret, as she would have done in a therapeutic group). The reason why she had to stop her visits naturally precluded conscious resentment; the group could not justifiably feel rejected or deserted in this situation. Nevertheless such resentment was of course felt, and showed itself in various ways. Once this was worked through, however, it became clear that the relationships established would not cease with the group meetings, and interesting and valuable developments took place.

It became clear that we could not expect Miss Brown to resume her regular visits, at all events for a long time, and gradually the members individually asked me to run a discussion group once a week. This would obviously be a different kind of group, but might help to preserve something of the work with Miss Brown. Although I was not at all sure how this could be achieved, eventually after a lot of thought I suggested that we should discuss a theoretical paper once a week. I hoped that by starting now from theory connected with regression and integration, we might in time meet the point reached with Miss Brown.

It became feasible to discuss involvement, with all the problems that this presents to individuals, because sufficient members of the team consciously experienced involvement themselves and were, therefore, able to conceptualize: they became able to make use of theoretical communications dealing with experiences which were so very real to them.

Perhaps the outsider who, like Miss Brown, makes an impact and evokes a response could be described as a thresholder, in the context of this paper: that is, someone who is able to help both insiders and outsiders by relating them to each other across the threshold of shared experience.

5
Role and function, 1962

The relation of assigned function to created role in a
therapeutic school for emotionally deprived children

*'Role and Function' was written at the request of Christopher Beedell, the
tutor of the advanced course in residential child care at Bristol University.
I read it to a large group of students and tutors at Bristol. The paper was
an attempt to communicate a realization which seemed to me to be at the
very core of all residential work with deprived children. I was also becoming
increasingly aware of the therapeutic potential amongst child care workers:
and of the tendency, in the Mulberry Bush and elsewhere in residential
boarding schools, for a split to occur between teachers and child care staff—a
split which could make therapeutic work impossible.*

Functions in any institution are essential: roles are inevitable.
Functions are usually clearly defined and accepted, whereas roles
may only exist by implication or may be denied or even forbidden.

You will be familiar already with the concept of roles and their
significance in group dynamics: here I shall only be considering
roles in relation to functions, especially in a context in which roles
and functions become incompatible. This is the context which
seems to me to present the crux of all difficulties in residential
work with emotionally deprived children.

I am especially indebted to Mrs Clare Winnicott for realizations
deriving directly from her valuable paper 'Casework and Agency
Function' (1962). I am also much indebted to Richard Balbernie,
whose insight and communications are woven into this paper;
and to the treatment team of the Mulberry Bush school, who
have so thoroughly discussed the problem of role and function
with me.

Mrs Winnicott writes: 'In functioning within an agency, a social
caseworker, as well as being a trained professional person who
uses her knowledge and skill to help people, also becomes something in relation to her clients on behalf of the whole community.'

People like ourselves, doing intensive work with emotionally deprived children, can only too easily slip, in the course of a therapeutic involvement with a child, (during a regression for example), into a state of isolation. This is rather an insulated child–adult cell which is unrelated to what (in our own case) is a complicated agency that travels out in ever-widening circles from the school to the parents or children's officers, the Board of Directors, the clinics, the local education authorities and the Ministry of Education. Should this insulation take place, as Mrs Winnicott goes on to say, 'We shall be failing our clients at the point of their deepest need, which is to reintegrate, through the services of the agency into the life of the community as independent self-determining people'. Such failure can result from an abandonment of function in favour of role, whereas I think that in therapeutic residential work both role and function are essential, and that it is usually possible for role to be contained within function.

The aim of the agency in relation to a residential unit must be to ensure continuity of function, which in our case means the provision of educational treatment. From an agency standpoint, a change of personnel (for example) must not affect the organization of the unit. It is often difficult, if not impossible, for an agency to tolerate a constellation of functions so flexible and interchangeable that there is little opportunity to establish a permanent nucleus of organization which can be clearly recognized and stated.

It is hard to describe the establishment in a therapeutic school. The presence of a teacher, a matron or a therapist may be confirmed, but confusion is likely to arise when further enquiry reveals that a teacher may sometimes cook a meal, a matron run a lesson group, a therapist clean paint and so on. This flexible function constellation is essential if provision of primary experience is necessary, and the agency is in a position either to support or undermine this flexibility.

Investigation of such overlapping and interchange of function shows that people doing this kind of work accept a function other than their own *in a particular context*. Sometimes such a context belongs to objective reality: a teacher may be ill, a matron away for a weekend. At other times, however, the context may be a matter of subjective reality, in which case one member of the team may take over a function other than his own in order to enable another member of the team to accept *a role*, created for him by the emotional needs of a child.

We have now reached a point at which we are thinking in terms of function in relation to role, rather than function in relation to agency.

It is clear that there must be continuity of function; what is not so clear is that there must also be continuity of role—that is, for as long as may be necessary in the treatment situation. People giving therapeutic help to emotionally deprived children must become involved with them in a way comparable to what Winnicott has described as 'primary maternal preoccupation'. Once this involvement has been launched, the most essential factor in treatment will be continuity of emotional provision. The task will now be to fill the gaps in the child's original experience in a way that can feel real to the child. This means that again and again it will be necessary for the therapist to 'hold a situation in time' as Winnicott describes mothers doing with their babies. Any gaps in such experience within an involvement will repeat the original disaster, and make it yet more difficult for the child to obtain further primary provision.

The actual temporary absence of the therapist is not likely to be as disastrous as anything which the child can feel as a withdrawal from commitment in the involvement. The most likely context in which this problem can arise is that to which I have already made reference, a situation in which role becomes incompatible with function.

Continuity—or rather the illusion of continuity—can only be achieved if there are supporters for providers, and providers for consumers. There may need to be much variety in the team constellation during a few hours in order to ensure continuity of provision for one difficult child. Nobody can achieve this continuity in isolation; there must be interdependence.

Mothers with infants need just this kind of support, and if they fail to obtain it from the environment they will not be able to provide for their babies; continuity of existence will break down and there will be gaps in their babies' primary experience. These are the gaps which we have to try to fill, in therapeutic involvement.

I would like now to consider some reality situations which have turned up in our particular school, when role and function have suddenly become incompatible and the involvement of grown-up with child has been threatened by the danger of interruption of continuity.

Robert was in a deep involvement, heading for a regression with his teacher Mr A, who was providing primary experience for Robert in a maternal role especially by accepting Robert's messiness and his blind panic rages.

On the occasion which I am about to describe, Robert was swept away by one of these rages during morning lessons. Mr A knew, because of the nature of the involvement and the very special adaptations which he needed to make to meet Robert's needs, that Robert would require to be alone with him for about an hour. However, the lesson group must continue to function. For Robert, Mr A was the only person at this moment who could contain him and his rage safely (Mr A had proved many times by then that he was able to do this).

Mr A was faced with a very difficult problem. He could have used his function (a teacher) as a defence, saying to himself, 'I am a teacher, I cannot allow Robert to behave in this way in my class.' Or he could have said, 'Someone else must take over Robert and see him through this rage—my function does not permit me to do so.' Or again he could have said, 'At the moment the needs of the group are more important than those of this particular child.'

I wish to consider these three possibilities before going further. Let us suppose that Mr A made the first response, saying 'I am a teacher . . .' In this case he would have to withdraw from the maternal role in regard to Robert and establish a gap between himself and the child by retiring behind his desk, and saying to Robert, by implication, 'I am your teacher, not your mother.' In this way he would be absolutely refusing the maternal role in which he had been created by Robert. Mr A would be making use of what I call a function defence, resulting in a breakdown of the continuity of involvement; in this symbolic way he would thereby be repeating just the kind of disaster which made a traumatic break in Robert's life as a baby.

If Mr A were to use the second response and were to say 'Someone else must take over Robert . . .' he would be handing over his therapeutic work to another person at the worst possible moment. Instead of containing this messy baby who looked like a ten-year-old boy, comforting him and cleaning him, he would from Robert's point of view be rejecting the baby because of his messiness—just when Robert needed him most.

Again, let us suppose that Mr A used the third response: 'The group's needs are greater than those of one child . . .' This might be true, but how could Mr A and the group know this? The evidence of Robert's breakdown into chaos would be there for both Mr A and the group to perceive: a rejection of Robert might be far more damaging to the group through their identification with Robert's needs, than their feelings of healthy resentment should Mr A sustain his maternal role. A child once said to me: 'Fair play is no use to people like us, because none of us want the same thing.'

Now in fact Mr A asked another member of the team, Mr B, to continue work with his group. Mr A literally picked up Robert and took him to a quiet place where the child could complete the panic rage in safety. In this way Robert obtained assurance of his own and Mr A's survival, and of Mr A's uninterrupted concern for him.

Mr B as supporter was *not* asked by Mr A to take over Robert, because the child could not be managed in the group. Mr B was in fact ensuring provision for Mr A and the group; he was not actually a teacher, his function was administrative so it could fairly easily be interrupted because it related to things rather than to people. Mr B would not be feeling that he had to take over the group because Mr A was unable to do something; on the contrary, he accepted the role in order to enable something to be done by Mr A—something which both Mr A and Mr B recognized as being of the utmost importance.

Mr A (the provider) had himself asked for help, and had been able to accept this help from the supporter, Mr B. At this moment Mr A created Mr B a supporter's role rather than seeing him in terms of his function as an administrator. Mr B's assigned function was sufficiently flexible to enable him to take over a group or do whatever else might be necessary in any specific context.

Mr B, however, in another context could himself be in need of help. For example, let us take a mealtime, when some child involved with Mr B having serious feeding problems could suddenly need to sit on Mr B's knee and be fed from a spoon. Now Mr B would give Mr A the role of supporter, so that Mr A would continue to supervise the mealtime while Mr B would be able to give the child involved with him the experience of being fed in a protected and containing situation. Of course there could be contexts in which neither Mr A nor Mr B would find it necessary to make the kind of adaptation to individual needs in a group which I have just described.

It is only during actual involvement that such continuity is essential–a recovering child can be scolded, sent out of class, or told to eat up his dinner–but an involvement is a slow and gradual process which must not and cannot be hurried or interrupted. It is the child–the consumer–who must set the pace, just as a baby does with his mother, and the provider who must judge what stage of the process has been reached.

Recently I found myself saying 'Mothers with babies should not cook omelettes!' You know how delicate and tricky is the art of omelette making; nothing must disturb the cook if the omelette is to be successful. Imagine an excited two-year-old, who has just found a tadpole, a buttercup or some such wonder. He comes to fetch his mother so that she can marvel with him, and she–because she is cooking an omelette–must say 'When I've finished cooking this, darling', and of course we all know that this will be too late. So, in my opinion, mothers of very little children should not cook omelettes or indeed anything unnecessary which cannot be interrupted by their baby's needs. In just the same way, when I am in an involvement with a disturbed ten-year-old, I must be able to break off from what I am doing so that I am there to meet *the child's creation of me.* Winnicott has written about this happening at the very beginning of life, and it turns up in just the same way in our work with older children.

The mother who has an organization built up round her baby, however practical and well-planned this may be, will not be providing what she and her child need; organization and ideas will have replaced orientation and experience. The mother who finishes an omelette, folds the ironing, and polishes that last piece of furniture while her baby cries in hope, then shrieks in anger and is finally silent in despair, will be leaving those gaps in continuity which result from premature failure in adaptation to her baby's needs.

We, if we allow orientation to go out of the window as organization comes in at the door, can repeat and confirm these gaps, so that the last state of the child may be even worse than the first.

If the agency assigns functions in an organization so rigid that it is impossible for roles to be contained and maintained within them, then the people in such an establishment may do all sorts of valuable work but they will not be able to make primary provision of experience. A built-in system of function defence will make continuity of emotional experience impossible, because this kind of system—however practical—forbids role acceptance, and witholds support of the kind I have been describing. What is even worse, the organization may try to cover the gaps, so that they will be hidden. There could be a proverb, 'Covered gaps make traps'. Rigid organization from outside can make individual and group integration unnecessary because high-powered organization can contain chaos. The greater the pressure of the chaos from within, the more rigid must the organization become; from such emotional environment springs riot, when the chaos finally breaks through the organization. This is true in individuals, in families and in groups. Organization needs to be built on the solid foundations of adequate primary experience, *when it will be appropriate and necessary*.

Of course, in terms of objective reality there will be many breaks in the continuity of provision in a therapeutic school. People will be having time off, may be ill for a time or away on leave. However, a child can keep things going in a remarkable way, as long as he is certain that the provider remains ready and willing to provide, and knows that he is failing the consumer. So long as the child is sure that the provider has not withdrawn concern there need not be a breakdown. Usually it is possible when necessary to maintain a lifeline of communication by letters, the telephone, and so on.

There is, as Winnicott has described (1958, p. 312) a great difference between 'failing' and 'letting down'.

So far I have described contexts where role and function have been fairly well established. Mr A was a teacher, and he was also

Robert's provider in a maternal role. Mr B was well aware of Mr A's function and of his role. Both Mr A and Mr B were experienced members of a team and used to this very special interdependence.

I now want to consider the kind of muddle which can come about so easily among people who are not accustomed to working in this way.

Miss M was a very gifted and sensitive student who was working with us at one time. She used to discuss her work with me quite frequently, and I am going to quote from my notes on one such discussion.

'One of Miss M's projects with us was a bedtime play group. This consisted of a small group of girls with whom she played and talked at bedtime, four evenings a week. This is the dormitory where there is a built-in dolls' house, which is kept locked up during the day at the request of the small girls themselves. Matron looks after the key and hands it over to whoever is with them when they want to use it.

'The first evenings which Miss M spent with this group she reported faithfully enough what she had observed, but found it difficult to actually *do* anything with the group. However, at the end of this first week something happened to her which seems worth reporting because of the implications in regard to training people to do this sort of thing.

'She was reading the little girls a story (she told me), everything was fairly peaceful, but she didn't suppose that she was doing very well. Another student—a man, older and more experienced than herself, who happened to be staying with us at the time—came into the room. She told me that she welcomed his arrival, and that things really happened in the group that evening, and he had helped her a lot.

'She described how all the children stopped listening to the story, and how in no time G had them all in a ring having a boxing match, and what fun this was for everybody—she could not get this sort of activity launched so successfully. She remarked that G (the other student) went out when it was time for the little girls to settle down, but they had taken a very long time to go to sleep and were very hostile to her, which puzzled her because they had had such a good time. At this point she could not find the key to the dolls' house, she looked carefully for it but it was nowhere to be seen. Eventually the little girls went to sleep.

'I asked her what happened about the key. She was very startled at my picking out just this from her report, as she regarded it as an unimportant detail, but nevertheless we found that she had not told matron about it, nor had she told the children that she had lost the key. As she spoke about it now to me she became more and more anxious; this was very different to the absolutely practical way in which she had reported its loss.

'I said eventually that I wondered whether the loss of the key had any connection with the arrival of G on the scene. She denied this vehemently, but when I said that I, personally, would be awfully fed up if someone came diving into the middle of my group, she said: "Well, although it was so nice to have him, it was a bit unsettling." I pointed out that G was unmarried, probably not at all used to little girls rushing around at bedtime, and the wholly feminine atmosphere that he came into at that moment might have felt a bit of a threat; what he did seemed to me to confirm this. Miss M said at once, "You mean the boxing?" I said: "Yes, the boxing . . . surely this was the kind of thing that might well go on with small boys in a dormitory in a prep school? I think he found it easier to think of them as small boys just at that moment." Miss M said, "And that's why they were so cross with me afterwards, because somehow they felt that I had let them down. I really should have sent G out, even if they were cross with me for doing so." I said that I thought she and the small girls must have felt rather invaded. G in fact had not supported the situation he found, because he was simply not able to do that then; he had created a situation of his own that was quite different from what he had found, but one in which he could feel safe.

'I asked Miss M whether now perhaps it became clear why she had lost the key, and she said suddenly, "Yes, of course I see, I was saying it is no use shutting the door to make things safe for the group, because someone will break in. I lost the key to the dolls' house to show what I meant to say, that it is no use locking up the dolls' house because somebody would break the lock if I did."

'We agreed that it was dreadful to be so vulnerable, but that this is the kind of thing that happens, and that understanding about it makes it easier. Miss M said, "Yes, if that happens again I think I shall ask G not to come in just at that time; or anyhow, if I didn't do something about that I would know why I was upset, and why the children were upset afterwards." Following this experience, Miss M became much more involved with the group, and her whole work took a step forward.'

Miss M had been created by the group of small girls in a maternal role. This was not so at other times, but belonged especially to bedtime. Her function was comparable to a supply housemother. Other people were involved with these five little girls, but as a group there was the beginning of something between them and Miss M. One could suppose that the story reading set-up gave her and the children satisfaction. She was able to feed them, and they to be fed by her.

G broke into this feeding situation; the breaking-in quality being determined by his inability to accept the role of supporter (the father containing and protecting the mother–baby set-up). G's function was even less clearly defined than that of Miss M; because he was only with us for a couple of days he was, for the most part, a fairly uninvolved observer, his time up to this moment had been spent among the older boys.

Miss M and the children, however, changed his role from a student observer into 'the father who looks after the whole family'. I suspect that G had a mild panic, and felt that he had disturbed the group. He was a bachelor, unused to babies, and may well have been alarmed by the totally female society in which he now found himself. He was well used to small boys and their ways, and at ease with them: in this emergency he created a role for himself (the big boy who plays with his small brothers, perhaps?) and launched the boxing match, thereby creating roles for the little girls (the small boys with whom he could play tough games) and a role for Miss M (the mother who cannot provide what boys need).

Of course G was not aware of all this, and neither—at the time—was Miss M, nor the children. Nevertheless they reacted to what was for them impingement.

Miss M became anxious and withdrawn, feeling inadequate and resentful in her role of a rejected mother. The little girls became excited and panicky. They were envious of boys, and here was a man who seemed to be assuring them that they could themselves be boys after all, while Miss M must now be the one who would be envious of them–she was now the only female in the group!

When G departed, Miss M tried to re-establish her function by looking after the children in a practical way. However, the little girls now felt let down; the bubble had been pricked and they felt disillusioned and angry with Miss M, who had failed to protect them against the seducing G. Miss M was feeling this herself, when she lost the key of the dolls' house.

G had unconsciously destroyed both Miss M's role and her function, because he had found it essential, because of his own panic, to create a role and function for himself which were *out of context* in terms of Miss M and the group.

Had G realized that he had no clearly defined role or function in this group, Miss M and the little girls would have created him out of their own needs a role as supporter and container. Unfortunately he was not able to allow other people to create him. There are many people–both parents and workers caring for children in any particular way–who create themselves and expect children to accept this creation. Although they may succeed in selling their self-creations, children dependent on them will find that they are unable to create these people in terms of their own special needs: the self-creation becomes a barrier against involvement, perhaps it may indeed be a defence against involvement. G may have been unconsciously afraid of what would be demanded of him if he allowed himself to be made use of. In fact, unless one is working with very mad children, adaptation can be remarkably localized; conscious involvement is only seriously inconvenient now and then.

You can see from the experience of Miss M just how confused functions and roles can become, and how essential it is that there should be empathy and interdependence between members of a team.

Another essential factor will be adequate intercommunication amongst the team, without which interdependence would be impossible. For such intercommunication to be possible there must be considerable insight; members of the team need to be able to experience, to realize experience and to conceptualize realization into a form which can be communicated. What happens all too often is that people start off with off-the-peg concepts and try to reach back to experience. A treatment team, working closely together in terms of role and function, by experiencing, realizing, conceptualizing and communicating can remain reliable, flexible and interdependent.

There are great difficulties, however, in establishing and maintaining communication and mutual understanding between the therapist who accepts roles and the agency that assigns function. Agency can be in touch with function which is relatively constant, function can be in touch with role providing there is flexibility such as I have been describing; but for agency to be in touch with ever-changing roles is out of the question. The most that should be expected of the agency is an orientation towards function interchange and role acceptance in principal.

One could compare this orientation with that of society's attitude in relation to a family constellation containing a mother with a new baby, when in normal circumstances the father is assisted by everyone in the environment to protect the mother–baby unity against impingement. Fathers are people who can usually exchange functions and take over roles for short periods–changing nappies, or cooking, or just comforting in the way that mothers do.

There are, however, many residential establishments (schools, hospitals, and so on) familiar to agencies where rigid organization and fixed function are firmly entrenched. There are many families where this is equally true; where organization has contained confusion, more or less successfully. Adults with this kind of background, functioning in an agency or in a function constellation in a residential unit, may well find that interchangeable functions and role acceptance with support are intolerable concepts, because they themselves may depend upon organization for survival and may have used 'function defence' to avoid role acceptance in family life.

I have talked a lot about the need for role acceptance. There is also the question of role refusal, which can be appropriate in certain circumstances.

There is really no need for a grown-up to accept a role from a child if they involve areas for the provider which are right outside his assigned function; role acceptance would then be courting disaster. It should only be occasionally that incompatibility of role and function presents problems; a role should usually be maintained within the scope of a function, otherwise continuity can only be assured at the cost of disturbing the psychic equilibrium of the group by too great and too constant demands for support being made by the provider, or by the provider stealing part functions.

For example: supposing a matron is involved with Tommy, a non-reader. She may well allow him to practice his reading curled up in a chair in her room and may support and encourage him in his efforts to read. It would be a different matter if she decided to teach him herself—perhaps by other methods than those used by his teacher. This would both interfere with her assigned function, because she would in any case not be able to maintain a providing role in an educational field and still sustain her own function, and furthermore, she would be stealing a part of the teacher's function thereby creating obvious problems for Tommy. She might well ask for and receive support from other members of the team in order to enable her to make this adaptation (unless the implications were clearly understood), so that a point could be reached that was comparable with giving support to a mother who was trying to put her baby to bed in the middle of Piccadilly Circus! Nobody has any right to accept a role which is going to put a prolonged and severe strain on function constellation or agency, nor should this be necessary. There are many symbolic ways of maintaining *created roles within assigned functions*.

I give an example of this in Chapter 9, where I describe walking up the village with a ten-year-old called Marguerite, who I knew needed to be picked up and carried home like an exhausted baby (Marguerite was in a regression at the time). I was wondering how I could possibly make such provision for her, when I found that at that moment she laid her hand in mine so that I could *carry her hand*, as though this were the whole child.

Apart from other considerations there is always the problem of time: a role accepted today may need to be maintained for a week, or a month or a year. It is necessary to localize adaptation in order to assure continuity in a therapy of primary provision.

When working with what I call 'frozen' children, I think it is important both to refuse roles and to use a function defence in order to preserve one's boundaries, and to make the child aware of the existence of these boundaries. 'Frozen' children are those without identities who attempt to merge with their environment in an effort to remain in a symbiotic state. It is very difficult to give help to such a child to enable him to progress to integration, rather than becoming a host, as it were, for his parasitic merger. One can, when working with these children, confuse collusion for delinquent ends with involvement for a therapeutic purpose.

Recently I had an interesting experience with such a child, a nine-year-old called Tim. He gave me a picture he had just painted, casually and with a charming smile, as we passed each other: children often give me pictures in this way, and my acceptance is usually all that is needed in the particular context. With Tim, however, I felt it wiser to ask: 'Will you tell me about it, Tim, before I let you give it to me?' It turned out that the picture was of a pirate ship (disguised) on its way to an island to dig up stolen treasure which was buried there. I was being invited to join the expedition and to have a share of the stolen treasure; had I accepted the picture I would also have been accepting the invitation. In fact, I refused the picture (giving my reasons), and Tim was able to make good use of my refusal to become a pirate.

SUMMARY

I have tried, in this paper, to put before you some ideas about the relation of roles to functions in a therapeutic school: much remains to be considered. However, I am going to attempt to draw my ideas together at this point.

Function and role must be present in any residential unit or agency. Where children are more or less integrated, and primary provision is not needed, function assigned by agency is as it were in the ascendancy: role will exist, but in a latent rather than a manifest form, and is unlikely to interfere with function or agency.

In a unit catering for severely emotionally deprived children in need of primary experience the situation must be quite different. Here, agency assigns function, but needs to be orientated to role acceptance within function. When role becomes (in a particular context) more important than function, the orientated agency is now able to allow interchange of function in order to assure continuity of role, when therapeutic involvement has become a subjective reality in treatment.

One might perhaps say that in the primary unity of a mother and her newborn baby, a super-ego is absent from the situation. The father and the supporting social environment protect the unity from impingement of super-ego forces. This frees the mother to be more or less completely preoccupied with her baby, relieving her of responsibility in all other fields, until she and her baby are ready to separate out into two individuals. Similarly, in the treatment of emotionally deprived children, the agency (representing society) allows the function (representing the father) to free role (representing the mother) to maintain the phase of involvement which must occur in a therapy of primary provision.

Occasional breakdown of therapeutic involvement is inevitable, but should this disaster happen frequently through lack of support, both agency and function constellation must take responsibility for a policy which is likely to cause further primary deprivation *within* a treatment setting.

The provider must whenever possible make provision through highly localized adaptation within function. When, however, role and function become incompatible in a particular context, the provider has a right to expect support from function and acceptance from agency.

6
The possibility of regression in a structured environment, 1963

These notes were written during a difficult time, when it seemed that the Mulberry Bush would have to be turned from an organism into an organization. I was attempting to adjust to changes which I found intolerable. This paper was an attempt to come to terms with a deeply altered emotional climate. These were problems for everyone concerned with the Mulberry Bush during this phase of development, many of which have now been resolved.

The provision of primary experience must depend on the insight and skill of the individual therapist, and on his or her capacity to be able to be sufficiently involved with the child to produce an emotional climate comparable to maternal preoccupation (I shall be discussing the nature of this 'climate' later). Furthermore, the therapist will need to be able to make appropriate adaptations to the child's special needs in this setting; these adaptations being provided with concern, consistency, and continuity over perhaps quite a long period of time. Such adaptations are symbolic, but essentially something *done* by the therapist for the child, or something *given* to the child by the therapist. What is done or given must be real (Sechehaye, 1951, talks of 'Symbolic Realization'). One says of justice: 'It is not enough for justice to be done–it must *be seen* to be done.' Of this primary provision through symbolic adaptation one could say: 'It is not enough for it to be done–it must *be felt* to have been done.' That the adaptation should feel right is as essential for the therapist as it is for the child (in this context 'the therapist' may be anyone in the place who is caring for the child).

Let me make it clear that I can imagine nothing worse than a conceptualized system of adaptation dosage, however well planned. One sees such a system employed by obsessional mothers with their babies. Many childhood psychoses have such a history: the mother claims with absolute truth, 'But I did everything I was taught to do for my baby.'

Clearly, therefore, provision of primary experience has to be made as the result of a slow and natural process between grown-up and child. It must be highly personal and individual; dependent – just as with a mother and her baby – on the particular personalities and the emotional climate in which the process takes place.

I have written elsewhere (Chapter 5) about assigned function and created role: the assigned function is the particular 'job' done by a person in a place, e.g. a teacher or a matron. The created role cannot be defined in terms of objective reality; indeed, such a role may never be recognized or stated: nevertheless, whatever the assigned function may be, every grown-up in the place will be created subjectively in many roles by both children and fellow workers.

When one comes to consider role and function in connection with primary experience, one sees at once that a grown-up therapeutically involved with a child can only hope to provide primary experience if he or she accepts a provider's role, within the assigned function. The narrower and more specific the function, the more difficult will it prove to provide the continuity of experience and meet the expectation of adaptation to needs, which is required by the child.

A mother who hands over her baby to various people in the course of twenty-four hours, or who goes out to work for long periods, will never establish such continuity: this is in fact just the kind of mother who is likely to have an emotionally deprived child, a child who has *gaps in his emotional experience* – unless someone else in the environment has taken over the provider's role in the original situation. .

In the same way, a person working in a place for a few hours every day, or all the time in a very specific context, may become involved with a child who is in need of 'gap filling'; but he or she may be unable to find any way of making continuous emotional provision which will 'keep the child going' and be sufficiently reliable to prevent further gaps in the child's life. A teacher, for example, in a boarding school for deeply disturbed children, who never gives a child a meal, or puts him to bed, or takes him out alone, has a much narrower field of provision and continuity open to him than would be available to him if he were to be in touch with the child outside as well as inside the classroom.

In our particular school there had been in the past extreme flexibility of function by grown-ups accepting provider roles. However, in our own case, flexibility was by no means successfully equated with efficiency, and the school was in no ordinary sense an efficient organization. (I must note here that now in 1967 I think we can claim to have achieved a flexible organization within which regression can take place without too many problems.) The same grown-up might teach a child, take him to the dentist, give him a bath, or paint a picture with him; the same therapist might ask the matron to treat a minor injury, take a child to the staff house and cook a meal for him. The therapist might spend money on a child (buying a symbolic gift of special sweets or some other special food) without making any formal arrangement in advance. He might ask another member of the team–on the spur of the moment–to take over his group for an hour or more so that he can free himself to see a child the whole way through a rage. Anybody, working in this way is continually 'committed beyond his capacity', as has been so well stated. I do not believe that adequate provision of primary experience can be made without such commitment. 'Localization' would seem to be the only possible solution, if the environment is to be as structured as most places really seem to need to be, and this is the theme which I wish now to discuss.

I would like to consider the particular problem of giving one small boy, Tommy, what he needed at one point in his treatment. Here is an extract from a letter from Tommy's mother.

Tommy has had no tempers, he has been quite good really. For the first four weeks at home Tommy only had about four nights' sleep, he used to lay awake all night long, and he never slept in the day. And he used to wet the bed and wet himself, or dirty himself. But he has not done that for the past three weeks. When he first came home I could not send him out to play, as he used to try and strangle the children he was playing with, and he started to talk like a baby. But he has stopped that now. But he won't wash or bath himself, and he won't comb his hair. He used to bath and wash, and comb his hair, but not since he has been home. He takes two hours to wash, and then someone has to wash him after because he has not really washed, just been playing about. He won't undress himself, or get dressed— but I make him do it . . .

My reply to this letter was:

Thank you very much for your letter which told me so much about Tommy during these holidays.

I can see how difficult it must have been for you to manage him at this stage, and in some ways I would have thought it better for him to have reached this stage at the Bush. However, in other ways it seems to be extremely important that he should have happened to have been on holiday and that he has been able to go through this with you in his own home—because this is where it all belongs.

What I feel you have described is Tommy as a baby again, because it seems clear that this is how he has behaved, and that his needs have been those of a baby. An experience such as this with you at home will make it possible for him to make more progress with us this term, because he has really gone back to the very beginning and filled in some of the gaps in the first year of his life—which you and I have talked about. I think he may do this again from time to time, both here and at home, and he was probably trying to do it towards the end of last term but was not able to because Mildred was going away.

You will remember we agreed when we met at the clinic that this was going to present real problems for him. What I think is going to be very important is that when we meet the behaviour you describe here—and when you meet it at home— we should all remember that this is a very little Tommy and not a big Tommy at all, and let him have the bit of babyhood experience he is asking for. Sometimes, of course, this may be too difficult, but whenever we can I think we should let him enjoy this. From experience with children who need this sort of thing I feel sure that this will help him towards recovery, in a way which nothing else can do.

I am hoping so much that you will come again to the Bush as soon as possible, so that we can talk about this together. I shall also be going to the clinic at some point this term, and perhaps we could meet again there.

I shall be seeing Tommy myself quite a bit this term, when he will obviously be missing Mildred, and will also, I know, be very unhappy at leaving you. . . .

You will now want to know something about Tommy. Perhaps he can speak for himself. Tommy had a song:

> The little boat sails
> On the water.
> And the little boat sails
> On the waves.
> And the little boat did
> And the waves was dead
> Then the waves had nothing
> To do with the little boat
> There was nothing for the little boat.

Tommy's song referred to his babyhood. He talked to me about the storm which had caused the waves which tossed the little boat about until they were dead and there was nothing left. What we reached later together was that there was once a time when the little boat was rocking gently on the calm and sunlit sea, before the storm. As Tommy said, 'I did not know there was a beginning to the song; it is like there being a nought before there is a one.'

I think all of us have unsung songs, unpainted pictures, and unwritten pieces of music inside us. The poets, the artists, and the musicians can communicate these in such a way that they sing, paint, or play their earliest experiences and find a response in us because we have also had a golden age at the beginning of our lives. But the disturbed children whom we try to help in our school have, all too often, no unsung songs within them. They have had nothing about which to sing.

It will be clear from her letter that Tommy's mother could not give him the regression he so much needed. It would really be more accurate to say that she was not able to allow *herself and Tommy* to experience involvement and commitment. She had not, however, shut her eyes to Tommy's needs: her letter was in a way an appeal for *us* to make the provision which she could not make in this context: any more than she had been able to do when (with Tommy three weeks old) she had handed Tommy over to a foster mother for nearly a year. How far, in the current structured environment (which must have resembled quite closely any good boarding school or children's home) could we undertake this provision for regression, which we were being asked to do by both Tommy and his mother?

There are several regression zones referred to in this letter.

1. Tommy lay awake all night. His mother—a reliable informant, on the whole—must have been awake herself, to know this. A child in regression will often stay awake at night in order to experience a continuity of care from the therapist, which is impossible during the busy day. For the grown-up involved this may mean a sleepless night spent by the bed of the regressed child, perhaps holding his hand, or in any case meeting his needs in a special way, for hours at a time.

2. Tommy's mother described him as being constantly wet and dirty. This, in a residential place, means an endless supply of clean laundry, with clothes changed every time the child becomes wet and dirty (just like changing babies' nappies) perhaps twice in a morning.

3. Tommy's mother referred also to Tommy's talking in a babyish voice. This would mean that if there was to be a regression the grown-up would have to respond in kind—at least to respond to unintelligible little noises, in the way that a mother communicates with her baby.

4. His mother described how Tommy would not dress or wash himself (remember this was a lively, active child), and if left to do so, took a long time. In treatment, if this zone was to be used, Tommy would have to be dressed and undressed unfailingly, perhaps for weeks on end.

There would probably have to be all sorts of secondary adaptations, but these were the regression zones indicated as appropriate by Tommy to his mother. She, unable to meet his needs, did all she could do by writing to me and passing on the necessary information (she had not often written to us, and never before in this way).

The problem now confronting us was just how to provide Tommy with his regression, in a structured environment, without dislocating a well-run organization which had only recently been established.

Let us consider the various points:

1. If a person in the place sat up all night (perhaps for many nights, and probably at least one each week), how could he or she work next day? Would all the other children in the place require this adaptation?
2. If Tommy was to be changed whenever he got wet or dirty, and was not scolded but comforted, how could the laundry be managed? And here again, surely all the other children would get wet and dirty too?
3. If Tommy's therapist responded to Tommy's baby talk it would often take some time to understand his communication. In the meantime, it might be getting-up time, lunch time, time for assembly, or time for lessons. The child and the grown-up would constantly tend to be out of step with the organization.
4. If Tommy was to be dressed and undressed every day by the therapist, this would cause disturbance to the established routine. Other children would say 'Why?' The grown-up concerned might well have some totally different function; he might be a teacher, for example. Perhaps he would not even be in the school at the particular time when Tommy gets up or goes to bed.

There is an Irish saying which goes roughly like this: 'If that is where you want to get to, you should have started from somewhere else', but this is a defeatist attitude. Tommy had to have his regression–and so did all the others like him–and the organization had to be preserved.

Sometimes a child at the Mulberry Bush uses sessions with me as a regression zone. Tommy did not do this, but he did bring a very small bear, which I gave him, to his sessions. He kept this little bear tucked in his pocket. This little bear was also Tommy– the little Tommy who needed the regression, who needed to be warm and contained and cared for. Tommy allowed me to help to take care of this little bear; one could call this localization of a kind, though displaced.

Tommy joined a spontaneous group which met in the evening with a member of the team. This group was making soft white toy rabbits, which became important in their creators' lives. Tommy made such a rabbit, to which he was devoted. A newcomer to the team, concerned for Tommy and knowing how easily possessions can be lost or destroyed, collected the rabbit from Tommy's bed one morning, and locked it up in the clothing store for safety. This was done out of kindness and concern, but Tommy was not able to understand this; regardless of all dangers, he wanted to look after his own rabbit. Finally, however, he settled for a compromise, by which he could see the rabbit from time to time. From a therapeutic standpoint such a compromise is unfortunately not satisfactory. Tommy had created the rabbit, which was therefore in the deepest sense his rabbit. Should he wish for his rabbit to be guarded, he could have asked the guardian of his choice. Children have in fact the right to lose what belongs to them. It can even be important for an emotionally deprived child to lose something he values; it may only be through loss that he can experience the realization that he now has something to lose. It is true that the rabbit could easily have been destroyed–perhaps even by Tommy himself–but there could be various important reasons for this to be a necessary experience. For example, he could be destroying something personal, and through this act he might have reached a feeling of *personal guilt* in respect of his destructive act, and an acceptance of personal responsibility for his actions.

One could say, of a more mature child, that the creation of the rabbit was more important than the actual rabbit.

–It would, however, be inappropriate to think of Tommy and other children who are so deprived, in these terms. For somebody like Tommy there is only the rabbit he imagines, and its magical projection into reality. The process of making the rabbit he would have found frustrating in the extreme, and this would be 'forgotten'; thus he preserved his infantile and magical omnipotence (the prototype of which was, he invented his mother and there she was!).

The rabbit might well–if it survived long enough–become a

transitional object, such as Winnicott has written about. For this to happen, the rabbit would need to belong completely to Tommy, rather than be looked after for him. We all know mothers who take such care of their children's toys that they can be proud of the toy's long survival. These, however, are not the toys which a child values: such toys are usually shabby, broken, and torn.

The little bear in Tommy's pocket was more localized than the rabbit. It was easier in a structured environment for the bear to become little Tommy than for the rabbit; grown-ups would not worry about a small bear in a pocket in the way they would worry about a rabbit on a bed.

Thinking on these lines, I find myself considering the letter from Tommy's mother. Tommy had attempted to have a regression at home, and this had proved impossible. The regression zones found by Tommy do not seem to be any more possible in a structured environment than at home. Symbolic objects like the bear and the rabbit remain once removed. We have considered the problems for the organization which would turn up if Tommy had a regression on his own personal lines (awake at night, wet and dirty, talking baby language, and refusing to dress and undress).

Nevertheless, without the regression Tommy could not make an emotional recovery. There is a real danger, however, that this kind of child may achieve a superficial social adjustment within the organization. This is what often happens in institutions of all kinds. Such children are emotionally impoverished when they grow up. Yet, for there to be a successful and smooth-running organization, there must be exact timing; rules and regulations must be kept. It is easy in such a situation for the child to prove that no special adaptations are available to him, and to withdraw from the possibility of regression.

I have spoken earlier of a very special emotional climate, which must exist if therapists are to provide primary experience. In the normal mother–baby unity there is no super-ego factor present; there is no feeling of guilt in respect of deep involvement with another living being. The mother who is preoccupied with her baby has projected all super-ego elements by whatever means at her disposal. The father then protects the mother–baby set-up from super-ego impingement. The therapist going into a regression with an emotionally deprived child must also project super-ego; furthermore, she must be supported in doing so (I would stipulate, however, that the grown-up must be fully conscious of the involvement, the projection, and the support given). This means that, just as the father protects the mother–baby unity from super-ego impingement (for example, dealing with the criticisms of envious relatives–'You are spoiling your baby' or 'You mustn't give in to him'); so, in the therapeutic involvement, there must be a supporting team or individual to say when necessary 'You are giving the child what he needs–go on.'

There are many factors in a structured environment which make involvement difficult. Rules and regulations, unless fairly flexible, can operate as stern super-ego demands, instead of being ego supportive. There is a time factor; a grown-up may be doing something very special for a child when a bell rings or a whistle is blown, and the grown-up realizes that he or she may actually 'get the child into trouble' by making him late for a meal. So the primary experience–whatever form it may have taken–may be interrupted: this interruption is in a subjective sense *for ever*, and is a faithful reproduction of just the kind of traumatic break expected by the child.

It is easy too for involvement to be seen as perverse. A man accepting a maternal role created by a small boy may look after the child in a maternal way. The fact that he is quite aware of what he is doing, discusses his work in detail, and so on, may not save him from suggestions that he is a homosexual. There is nothing more vulnerable than a therapeutic involvement: once guilt has been let in at the door, primary preoccupation flies out of the window.

I have described some of the difficulties likely to turn up in a structured environment when a child needs a regression, and some of the reasons for these difficulties. We are left with the question: given these circumstances and accepting the need (provisionally, at all events) for a highly structured environment, how could Tommy's needs be met?

I have suggested localization (in other papers I have referred to the successful use of localizing symbolic adaptation). Such an approach is of course open to all sorts of abuse. Arbitrary, adult-determined adaptations, even though based on Tommy's reported expectations, would not 'feel right' to either grown-up or child; they would only, at best, appear to be therapeutically correct techniques. Here again, we all know the mothers who do this sort of thing because it is all they can do: we also know the devastating effect this has on the babies.

Localized adaptation, therefore, needed to be selected and indicated by Tommy himself. Let us look again at the total requirements.

1. Someone with him at night.
2. To be constantly wet and dirty and to be constantly made warm and clean.
3. To have baby talk accepted as a means of communication.
4. To be dressed and undressed.

Ideally, all this provision would need to be made by one person (I have done this myself quite frequently, so I speak from personal experience). In the absence of a provider, however, the child will accept a provider substitute (usually the person who specially acts as supporter to the involvement), but there must be a principal provider. The result would be a climate and environment capable of containing Tommy's regression. Let me be quite clear about this; it could not be provided within our organization, for perfectly good reasons. The organization could only be slightly disrupted, if at all. The regression had to be drastically localized.

Now it would be easy to say:

1. Someone – even Tommy's provider – could sit with him for ten minutes each evening.
2. Someone (it probably could not be the same person) could give him clean handkerchief tissues whenever he asked for them.
3. Someone could put on his tie every morning, or brush his hair, or do up his buttons, etc.
4. His own provider could accept baby talk from him in some special context.

Any of these adaptations might succeed, but only if, having failed to obtain the total regression, Tommy himself were to indicate the form of localization which would feel right to him; as long as this also 'felt right' to his provider, one could be quite optimistic. It was much more likely that the grown-up would say

'I'm sorry, Tommy, I can't dress you, but I will do up your buttons' or whatever. There would be a different state of affairs if the grown-up were to say 'I wish I could dress you, Tommy, but I have to do something else at that time' (or whatever the facts may be) 'perhaps you and I can find something I *can* do for you that'll feel right, and be what you need me to do. It's no use my saying I'll do something unless I really can.' Of course the grown-up concerned would say this in the kind of words which would be meaningful to the child; but this would be the content of such communication.

Sooner or later the child would then indicate the adaptation zone and the localized area within this, but the grown-up–the provider–would need to be sensitive and aware enough of the implications to understand and recognize such an indication.

For example: Peter came to me for sessions over a long period. He needed a localized regression for various reasons and had indicated several zones for regression which would have been impossible for me to use continually and reliably in the way he would need. He always seemed to have a running nose and to be miserable about it yet unable to find any comfort, so I took care of his nose over quite a long period. I brought handkerchief tissues, and when I was not there I let him know with whom I had left a supply for him. I provided a little pot of cold cream to soothe the roughened skin: in this was I able to take care of his nose and to show him how much I was concerned about him, even when not present. The hopelessly running nose was a signal which I picked up, and I really *did* mind about his poor nose; whatever we do for the child must *matter to us*.

This is why one cannot give instructions to people in a place; one cannot hand over therapeutic techniques in penny packets. This is as true for mothers and babies as it is for therapists and their patients. Mothers need to do what feels right to them and their babies. It is no use telling an obsessional mother to put her baby on a demand feeding regime: this will be alien to her, and if she carries out orders, she will do so in such a way that she and her baby will suffer.

Insight can only be gained slowly, and one must not confuse insight with intuition. People can only do therapeutic work in terms of themselves as they really are. We cannot teach this kind of work; we can only give people permission to learn, and support them in *meeting* the child's needs, when they realize what they really are.

The greatest obstacle to regression and to the provision of primary experience is the resistance to involvement. People can feel (or be made to feel) guilty in the way I have described; they are also usually unconsciously aware that involvement is a vulnerable, undefended, and dangerous state. For therapeutic involvement to be present there must be a supporting emotional climate, however structured the environment may be. Even in the case of the most localized adaptation, support will still be needed if the provider is to feel able to be sure that the provision is valuable and necessary.

I have discussed the possibilities of Tommy's regression, and it may interest you to hear the sequel to the correspondence I have quoted. I started writing this paper at the beginning of a term, and was surprised and impressed by just how well Tommy was tackling various difficult problems in the school, especially the departure of a much loved teacher. I have not mentioned before the fact that we had done a good deal of work with Tommy's mother, and that a lot of work had also been done for her before Tommy came to us.

Towards the end of the summer, there had been indications here that Tommy was 'asking for' a regression, and I had talked about this to his mother before he went home for the holidays. When I received the letter from her which I have quoted, it never occurred to me that she was asking my approval for what she had already done, rather than asking for my understanding that this was something she could not really allow herself to do. I did mention that she must have been awake herself at night in order to know that Tommy was not sleeping; imagine my surprise and delight when I had an interview with her at the referring clinic and found that in fact she herself had been able to provide Tommy with the total regression which had not been available to him here, the previous term. What is more, she was able to tolerate the thought that this had been a pleasurable experience to her.

She had moved Tommy into her own room, and had been awake with him all night, while he gazed out of the window and talked to her; she had taken off his wet and soiled clothes and had bathed and dressed him with clean clothes on every occasion when this was necessary; she had accepted his baby talk as communication; she had dressed and undressed him in the morning and at night, as though this was the most normal state of affairs: and she had done all this with feeling and insight. The psychiatrist supervising Tommy's treatment (who was with us), Tommy's mother and myself, were all equally happy as we talked about this. Tommy's mother knew that there were going to be more regressions, and was prepared to go through them with Tommy. There was still a need for localized regressions in the school, but the fact that Tommy was able to have a total regression with his mother, made these both less essential and easier to provide.

In this case, however, we had a mother who had gained insight through treatment and who had been given enough support by all of us to become involved with her own child. There are only a few mothers who can be helped in this way so that they can give the therapy themselves: there are the countless deprived children in need of a regression who are entirely dependent on the people who care for them in residential placement.

7
Problems of role acceptance, 1965

This communication is really a postscript to 'Role and Function', and was also read to the advanced residential course at Bristol University. It was based on discussions with Richard Balbernie, whose recently published book 'Residential Work with Children' (1966) will be essential reading for all those who work with deeply disturbed children in residential places.

In the course of trying to help emotionally deprived children of any age, one becomes accustomed to being created, annihilated, and re-created in terms of their particular needs at any given time. Since these needs arose in the first place through gaps in primary experience, such creation of the therapist is as a mother; this will be true whatever the real sex of the therapist may be. Obviously it is easier for a woman to accept this subjective creation, because for most women a maternal role is (at a conscious level, anyhow) acceptable. A man may find it very much more difficult to meet such needs, because of the threat to his masculinity and to his prestige as an actual or potential husband or father.

In normal family life, however, fathers are quite capable of being very good mothers in times of emergency; they can give feeds, change nappies, and manage babies extremely well: they often do so, should this prove necessary; and do so, furthermore, with pride and satisfaction.

Should mothers have to be fathers, even in comparable emergencies, there seem to be greater difficulties for mother and child; perhaps this is because a father's role at the very beginning is essentially protective of the mother–baby set up. As time goes on it is the father who interrupts this unity, in a very positive but disturbing way; so that for a mother to have to protect her own unity with her baby, or to interrupt this unity herself in the absence of the father, is to split her personality in a way which could be seriously damaging to herself and her baby.

People working with neurotics are dealing continuously with transference phenomena belonging to secondary experience following integration. The therapist may be playing the part of father, mother, brother, or sister; to say nothing of a grandparent; or indeed anybody who has played a significant part in the patient's development. If one is working with the emotionally deprived, it is likely that one will always represent (until integration) an aspect of the mother. When working with neurotics, the patient continues to know that one is not really his father, mother, or whatever, but that it feels to him *as if* this were the case. Emotionally deprived people – either grown-ups or children – leave out the 'as if': for them one *is* the mother. This type of transference has been called 'delusional'.

We who work with children and adolescents in residential places meet many more emotionally deprived children than neurotics. We have, then, the task of providing primary experience in symbolic form; the task of 'gap filling'.

In order to carry out this task we need support for the children and ourselves (comparable to that given by the father in the family situation), and I think this really does mean that one cannot do this work alone: there must be a person or a team to accept a paternal role in relation to the worker and child (whom I shall call the provider and the consumer). What often happens is that the organization, or current policy, or special circumstances, leaves out the paternal support: then the worker (man or woman) who has allowed the deprived person to have expectations from a 'mother' is suddenly unable to be a mother in context (i.e. at the right time and in the right place) so that the whole vital process breaks down. Every time this happens – and deprived people do go on trying to find what they need – it becomes more difficult for them to regress; their defences become more rigid; failed expectations change to compulsive demands; and premature disillusionment creates hard and cynical attitudes.

It is a sad fact that organization, in the ordinary social sense of discipline, ideas of fair play, and above all, certain moral assumptions, tend to bring about the breakdown of primary experience in residential places. There are many reasons for this: one may perhaps be that organization of a certain kind can be an elaborate defence against the possibility of regression. People have complicated feelings about regression, both in regard to the provider and to the consumer.

'They'–and by 'they' I mean colleagues, committees, inspectors, and so on–may say:

1. 'A seventeen-year-old should be on his own feet by now–he'll soon have to be out in the world.'
2. 'We won't have favouritism here.'
3. 'There's something kinky about a man looking after a boy as though he were a baby.'
4. 'It is quite wrong for a worker to spend so much time with one child.'
5. 'Each person has his own job here, and it would cause chaos if there were overlapping.'
6. 'Children should not be spoilt.'
7. 'Discipline must be maintained.'
8. 'The whole place will break down.'

These people may themselves be emotionally deprived and beyond hope of emotional provision. They therefore withhold and forbid the support which would make regression possible; as a result, men and women who are being good enough 'mothers' to deprived children and adolescents going through a babyhood process suddenly find that they have to become authority figures, interrupting the regression themselves. A process should never have to be terminated by an *act*: for example, weaning needs to be slow and gradual. They do not even become 'fathers' in order to meet the needs of the child, but to satisfy the demands of the organization. They say: 'I must stop taking care of you because it's time for something or other, and you must go somewhere or other', thereby destroying the unity of time and place (what Winnicott calls 'holding a situation in time'). One could say that they have to change from creative to anti-life activity as the result of inappropriate and external super-ego forces. They have to behave in a way which is inevitably over-determined because it is utterly alien to their intuitive or insighted awareness of emotional need.

Women in such circumstances deny their femininity, betray their creativity as mothers, and of course experience deep feelings of guilt because they have had to let down the person (grown-up, adolescent, or child) with whom they have become deeply involved, and for whom they may be at that time the only person in the world.

Men accepting maternal roles for therapeutic reasons can be forced into positions of authority, dealing out sanctions to the children for whom they have been providing babyhood experiences, because their maternal roles are resented.

It is as though people whose roles are broken into in this way become like tender, preoccupied mothers feeding and washing small babies, who must suddenly tell their babies, 'And now go and mix your feed, and wash your nappies . . .'. It is, of course, because of guilt that they react in this way: sometimes they hold their ground, and then there is trouble in store.

However, there are sometimes groups of people working together as a team with adequate 'agency' support who can, either spontaneously and intuitively, in such a manner that maternal roles can be maintained and supported. Paternal roles can come into the picture appropriately, in context, and in a way which is of real therapeutic value; helping rather than interrupting primary processes leading to integration as individuals.

This must all sound very theoretical, and you may feel—as in a way I do myself—that people should do this sort of thing naturally, and that there is a danger of intellectualizing, of falling over one's feet. However, I believe that it is important to know (to some extent, anyhow) what one is doing: working together on a basis of 'hunch'—what the Germans call *Fingerspitzengefühl* is not really sufficiently reliable, because this sort of co-operation depends too much on emotional climate and current mood. It is terribly easy to undermine a colleague's work through the use of intuition as a weapon: this can be done quite unconsciously in a moment of envy or anger. Once, however, one is consciously aware of what a colleague is trying to achieve through maternal or paternal role acceptance, there is much less risk of unconscious sabotage, and more likelihood of conscious and creative supporting role acceptance either by individual or group.

It is perhaps more difficult for women, working in a residential school or home, to allow men to care for children in practical ways which they may feel are their domain; to put a child to bed, for example, or to look after another who is sick, or do a little girl's hair.

Function can become a substitute for role; many people who are afraid of commitment refuse roles, and put all the feeling that would have belonged to the role in regard to people into the function in regard to things; like the kind of mother who is involved with her child's clothes, rather than with her child.

So far I have only spoken about people prepared to accept father and mother roles, and about some of the super-ego factors which are likely to weigh in against role reliability in residential places. Now, however, I want to turn to the very fundamental problem which turns up everywhere, even where roles *have* been accepted and supported. I refer to collusion, which I feel to be one of the most insidious hazards of residential work, or indeed of any work with emotionally deprived clients.

There is the overt type of collusion, which one can recognize without too much difficulty, in oneself and one's colleagues. For example, a man gets involved with an adolescent boy, which results in communication becoming established between them. Presently the boy brings accusations against another grown-up–a woman perhaps–a person whom the man does not like. Of course there is nothing wrong in the boy 'letting off steam' to this man whom he trusts; but if this man becomes identified with the boy in hatred of the woman, he is in a collusive position, identified as the father with the son against the mother. This is very different from a position of empathy, where the man is trying to understand the boy's feeling of hate for the woman, without such identification taking place. This example is of a relatively superficial kind of collusion; a man and a boy merged in hate (and probably some envy) of a woman (envying her because she is a potential mother who can have a real baby).

I have been having informal discussions for some time with the devoted parents of a very disturbed adolescent patient, a boy. The father of his family has many of the qualities which go to make an ordinary devoted mother; he has a deeply feminine part of himself of which he is quite unconscious. In order to keep this part hidden, he has to shut off a part of his personality at great cost to himself, presenting a pseudomasculine attitude which is over determined and really alien to him. For example, he is authoritarian and punitive on occasion to his son, in a way which is very unreal.

His wife, who is very beautiful, intelligent and talented, is in fact masculine behind the feminine facade of charm and beauty: the children in this family have been seriously damaged by the interminable conflict between the girl part of the father's personality and the boy part of the mother's personality. The collusion in this case is between the son and the boy part of the mother, against the feminine part of the father. This is one aspect of a complex picture, but I am only concerned here with suggesting that unconscious components are present all the time, bedevilling conscious aims and tending to produce a crippling undertow.

Collusion with delinquents can be present without anyone quite knowing how this has come about. Delinquents are seductive and skilful, and should be able to rely only on our continued concern. Involvement with them becomes merger, and once this has taken place the therapist is no longer in a position to help his client.

A student recently gave me an interesting example of such a delinquent trap. She was playing hopscotch with a small boy, and the game was proceeding quite normally when she made some mistake. The boy said at once, 'That's all right, we won't count that against you.' She accepted this gesture as kindness and concern, until she found that he was now cheating and ignoring the rules: when she protested he looked surprised and said, 'Well, you cheat too.' This was collusion through role acceptance, the role being that of another delinquent boy.

I myself had an interesting experience of this kind (which I have also described elsewhere in another context) with a 'frozen' delinquent who was just starting to feel guilt and conflict. He wished to give me a picture he had just painted; he was in rather a hurry, as we passed each other in the passage. The picture was of a sailing ship on a smooth sea; the sun shone, seagulls flew round the masts, and all looked tranquil. However, before I accepted this picture I asked the boy to tell me about the ship. He was a trifle reluctant to do so, saying: 'It's a picture for you.' At length, however, he revealed that this was a disguised pirate ship on the way to find some stolen treasure, hidden previously on an island. I was to be involved in this adventure, to be one of the crew, and to have some of the stolen treasure. When I refused to accept the picture or to have anything to do with the pirates or the treasure, the boy was very angry; he tore up the picture and stamped off. Had I accepted the male role of a pirate seeking stolen treasure with him, I would have accepted a role which would have made it impossible for me to help him: in accepting the picture I would have unwittingly accepted the role. Here I would have been trapped into a male delinquent role, which would have hopelessly undermined the maternal ego-supporting position which I held.

Experiences have formed our egos: it is our fathers and mothers who have given us their experiences so that they have become part of us. Men have creative maternal corners tucked away in unexpected places: women have male paternal sides of which they may be unaware. Intuitively, our customers for emotional experience will find these bits of us—and sometimes bits we ourselves do not know about. It is just these unknown nooks and crannies which cause complications in the counter-transference. Whatever turns up in this way is worth looking at and sometimes understanding; then we can be in a position to make use of more of ourselves and to allow our clients to do so. We shall also be in a better position to judge whether we should accept or refuse the male and female roles assigned us in the course of our work; and be less likely to drift into collusion, which can only sabotage ego growth in our clients and ourselves.

8

Helping other people to help us, 1965

I read this paper to a refresher course for child care workers. It was at this point that I became more aware of the tremendous therapeutic potential in the field of child care. The questions and comments of my audience made me feel very close to them, and I enjoyed this experience deeply.

Students inevitably assign us parental roles; the nature of such roles depends on the student's own history. Because we are expected to assign and supervise their work, and especially because we are the people who take ultimate responsibility, there is quite enough in the situation to make it easy for them to continue to treat us as parents. This tends to push them into a sibling relationship with the babies or the children involved; the nature of this relationship will again depend on their experiences or lack of experiences with brothers and sisters.

Students may still be in adolescent doldrums, and in any case are likely to be coping with some problems belonging to their own babyhood and early childhood, which are sure to turn up in relation to any older people with whom they come in contact. This is precisely why I think problems are inevitable, and this is also why we find it difficult to help them to help us. This is especially true if the students are in any way themselves emotionally deprived; when they are certain to be over permissive or over-authoritarian, depending on whether they are wanting to give the babies everything they themselves need, or out to prove that the babies cannot have what they themselves lack (one sees both extremes in deprived parents).

Students may need to be good, ideal mother figures in the children's lives, and at the same time good, ideal children in our lives. So much goodness is very hard to tolerate—one may feel terribly bad oneself compared to the students—the children say how nice the students are (the implication being how nasty we are). It can be difficult to realize that we have been made into convenient bins to contain the badness which the students are disowning. For example: a child may ask a student for another cake or a sweet, and the student may reply: 'I'm not allowed to give you any more, so-and-so would be cross with me', instead of taking the responsibility as a grown-up of saying 'no'; the student has thus turned us into forbidding parental figures—for themselves as well as for the children. Of course this is not conscious, and sometimes one cannot make out why one feels irritated by these young people, who are always so friendly and nice and never seem to get tired, cross, or frustrated.

Recently we had living with us in our own home (for a year) a young psychologist from abroad who was learning psychotherapy; I am going to call her Zoe. I supervised Zoe's work with a child who was in treatment with me, and several times each week we met together to discuss her experiences. Zoe has given me permission to talk about some of these experiences, because we both feel that they are interesting, and that the episodes which I shall be describing illuminate the particular problems of student and supervisor in any residential work.

Zoe was in fact a very normal and intelligent person, of great integrity and sensitivity, yet even so there were serious difficulties in the situation for both of us, which we tried to tackle together.

Lucinda was a delightful and intelligent child who was living with us during her treatment, which was needed because of serious emotional problems arising from her first year of life. She has made a remarkable recovery.

Remembering Lucinda's violent reaction to newcomers, I tried to prepare Zoe for what was to come; I explained that this charming little girl was capable of most subtle manipulation, and in particular was able to create discord by playing off one grown-up against another (just as she did with her own family).

I have found that it is valuable to concentrate on a particular *situation* for discussion. I have come to regard a situation as something very exact. For example, I suggested initially to Zoe that we should only talk about Lucinda's bedtime—from the moment that Zoe called her for her bath till she was tucked up in bed and ready to go to sleep. However, for various reasons this did not prove to be a successful choice of situation (partly because I had been putting Lucinda to bed myself for a long time) so we thought again and decided on a walk–after tea–between five and six o'clock. I explained to Zoe that I was not looking for a list of accurate observations of Lucinda's behaviour, but rather for descriptions of actual experiences which she and Lucinda had together in the course of the walk, which we could then talk about.

Here are some of the situations, the first of which happened before the walks, just after Zoe's arrival.

Situation 1. Lucinda scratched her finger very slightly, and Zoe offered to treat the scratch. Lucinda said that she did not know where the first-aid equipment was kept. Zoe offered to wrap the finger up with paper, and Lucinda accepted this offer. However, it then became apparent to both of them that the paper must be tied onto the finger. Zoe asked, 'Have you a piece of string?' and Lucinda said, 'There is some in Mrs D's room' (our bedroom). She went into our room and brought a piece of string from my workbasket. Zoe tied this round the paper, and Lucinda then said, 'This will be a secret between us–don't tell Mrs D, she'll be angry with us for taking the string from her workbasket in her room.' At first Zoe agreed to keep the secret, then she had misgivings and told Lucinda that this was not a secret which she could keep, but that she was sure that Mrs D would not be cross–would Lucinda tell Mrs D herself? Lucinda agreed.

Later Zoe told Lucinda that she had told me about the string, and Lucinda's response was: 'Well, that's two people who've told her, I'd already told her myself.' In fact, she had said nothing to me.

This lacks the precision of a planned situation, but it is easy to see in this story the theme of manipulation and collusion which could so easily have put Zoe in a false position, and could have made real communication between us impossible. Lucinda turned me into a threatening authority figure, dangerous to herself and to Zoe. Zoe lost ground by agreeing in the first place to keep Lucinda's secret, but did not continue to collude, although her refusal made Zoe less 'good' in Lucinda's eyes. This was difficult for Zoe because Lucinda obviously liked her and was being very charming to her.

Situation 2. The walk plan was launched. Lucinda returned from school and had tea, then she and Zoe set out for a walk. Zoe suggested that Lucinda could choose which way to go. Lucinda said: 'I know a nice way to go', and they set out together across the fields. Presently Zoe became aware that Lucinda was taking her to the Primrose Wood; for various good reasons no one was allowed to go there without our permission, and Lucinda knew this. Zoe refused to go to this forbidden wood, and met Lucinda's anger.

Zoe and I had by now discussed collusion, and she was able to see how easily Lucinda could destroy our relationship; just as she had nearly destroyed her father's second marriage, and had, in the course of treatment, tried to come between my husband and myself in the same way.

Situation 3. There had been a heavy fall of snow, so Lucinda chose to make a snowman, as part of the walk. At first, in all situations, Zoe found she was being told what to do by Lucinda, and was carrying out her commands. Now, however, when Lucinda told her, 'You are to make the arms', Zoe felt acute resentment and said that Lucinda could do this herself. Lucinda was furious.

Zoe was able to realize that Lucinda was using her as though Zoe was just part of herself; something of which Lucinda could make use. Zoe sensed the ruthless quality of Lucinda's behaviour, and did not have to feel guilty about her resentment, which was appropriate.

Situation 4. Lucinda was so angry at not being able to control and direct Zoe on another walk, that she went off alone in a rage.

Situation 5. Zoe took Lucinda for a walk, and initiated a discussion as to the aim of this particular expedition. Lucinda said, 'You decide where we'll go.' However, she then turned down any suggestions made by Zoe. Finally they set out. There were still patches of snow on the ground; they came to such a patch of snow, which was (to quote Zoe) 'very white and fine'. Zoe exclaimed, 'How beautiful that is!'–whereupon Lucinda immediately jumped on it with dirty boots. Zoe protested indignantly, saying, 'You've spoilt it!' and at once Lucinda tried to cover up what she had done, and smooth the snow on top. Zoe said, 'Now it's all right.'

When we came to talk over the situation it was difficult for Zoe to see that her reassurance to Lucinda took away from the child an opportunity to accept personal responsibility for a destructive act. The reassuring 'It's all right' came because Zoe herself felt anxious; she did not wish to face this destructive part of Lucinda, and identified with Lucinda in 'covering up'–literally–the destruction.

On the same walk–i.e. within the same situation context–Zoe and Lucinda went onto some land which could have been private, in order to feed some cattle with grass (the cattle were in enclosures). Lucinda was anxious and asked constantly, 'Is it all right?'

On the way back she agreed with Zoe that I should be consulted about feeding cattle on this bit of land, but Lucinda kept saying, 'We didn't harm them, did we?' Zoe again gave reassurance, but when we talked about this we decided that Lucinda was not only talking about the feeding of the cattle, but also about the snow episode. She also made Zoe anxious in case they had in fact trespassed. Zoe told me at once about all this, but had she not been able to let me know at once what had happened she might have felt very worried.

Situation 6. During this discussion about Lucinda and the snow, Zoe began to see the connection between this story, and another earlier occasion which she now remembered. This had been on a walk after heavy rain. Zoe told Lucinda not to go into puddles. Lucinda did so, pretending not to hear. Zoe found she could not insist because *she herself liked to go in puddles!*

This brought us to the whole question of responsibility: after all, Lucinda was in our care. Where did Zoe's responsibility begin and end? In a way, because my role in regard to Zoe was that of supervisor, I was certainly to some extent responsible for Zoe as well as for Lucinda. We came to the conclusion that Zoe's responsibility was that of any grown-up in relation to a child. She had to accept her grown-upness as compared with Lucinda's childhood. If she could do this successfully she would not have to wonder so much about 'Yes' and 'No', and she would be much less likely to collude.

As Zoe became more reliably established as a grown-up,

Lucinda went to great lengths to draw her back into collusion. Usually Zoe found it possible to recognize these attempts and maintained her position as a reliable grown-up, able to say 'no' on occasions without fear of Lucinda's hate.

Lucinda became less enthusiastic over the 'walk situation'; originally she was able to feel that Zoe would be entirely under her control, now as it became evident to her that Zoe could no longer be manipulated she started to behave in a different way.

Situation 7. Lucinda said that she could not put her boots on: she said to Zoe, 'There is a spider in my boot—you must shake it out and put my boot on, I'm too frightened.' Zoe assured her that she would wait for her, but that she was sure Lucinda could cope with the boot; there was a lot of fuss and stamping about, and presently Lucinda was ready to set out. Lucinda tripped and nearly fell at a particular place on the walk, and Zoe noticed that this was connected with refusals to be bullied by Lucinda. Lucinda said, 'I wonder why I always fall at that place.'

Sometimes Lucinda was now actually unwilling to go on the walk! On one such occasion she fell down and grazed her knees. She could only enjoy a situation which was completely under her control. However, at the same time she seemed to be beginning to enjoy herself in a new way. She would dance along, and sing songs of her own about the sky and the trees, in a very spontaneous and free way.

Talking about this, Zoe and I felt that Lucinda was now more secure because Zoe was looking after her; this was because it was a walk for a grown-up and a child, rather than for two children.

However, Lucinda was at pains to show that she was not dependent on Zoe; seeing hoof marks on a lane she claimed that she knew the rider (a grown-up lady) very well. They passed a farmer who said 'Good evening' to them. Again Lucinda claimed that she knew this farmer very well, and that that was why he had said good evening.

On the whole, Lucinda was now much more relaxed on the walk, and did not seem to have the same desperate need to control the situation.

Recently an episode happened outside the walk situation, but which seems to me typical of how things can go wrong for even the best of students, through no fault of their own.

Someone found an invitation for Lucinda, to a children's party, under Lucinda's bed; this must have been there for some time, and the date was for the very next day. I talked with Lucinda about this: she went round and round in verbal circles–she had forgotten, had meant to tell me, and so on. I reminded her of other occasions when she had done this sort of thing to us and to her parents; she would go to school next day and say: 'Mrs D hadn't time to do anything about it, so I can't come to your party!' Eventually we sorted her out and Lucinda decided it would be more fun to go to the party than to be persecuted by me.

I asked Zoe if she knew anything about all this, and found, as I had expected, that Lucinda had told her about the invitation, saying that she was not sure yet whether or not she would be going. Zoe had thought I knew, so had not mentioned the matter to me.

We discussed how matters would have turned out if the invitation had not been found under Lucinda's bed, and we were then able to see that Lucinda would not have gone to the party. She would have told Zoe, or allowed Zoe to think, that I had not made the necessary arrangements: Zoe would then have been identified with Lucinda in establishing me as a persecutor (i.e. the person who doesn't take trouble). Had the invitation not come to light, I might *never* have known what had happened. There would, however, have been a barrier built by Lucinda between Zoe and myself. I am sure that it is the presence of such unknown barriers between students and ourselves which can make work very difficult for them and for ourselves.

Lucinda is still someone who finds it difficult to love and hate the same person; to find a person good and bad, rather than all good or all bad. She herself sometimes feels all good and sometimes all bad.

Because she needs someone who is all good, there must always be such a person in her environment; but this means that there must also be an all bad person, so that she can only love one person and only hate another: her aim is to keep her two people away from each other. In order for Zoe to be all good, I had to be all bad; indeed, during the experiences I have been describing

Lucinda treated me as though I was a wicked witch, the Queen out of 'Snow White' or just her own stepmother! I could stand her hatred of me, and not feel too bad myself, only because I understood a little of what was going on between Zoe and Lucinda. Zoe, through her understanding, was able to refuse the 'all good' role, and Lucinda became much more real and more able to love *and* hate both Zoe and myself (i.e. I became less bad, and Zoe became less good from Lucinda's point of view).

I think that it is very difficult to tolerate this sort of experience; when a child for whom one has cared devotedly for a long period suddenly treats one like a monster, whilst treating some young stranger with praise and love. However, very often the story between the lines is similar to what Zoe and Lucinda went through.

Perhaps it helps one a bit to realize that Lucinda was not consciously doing these awful things, and that Zoe was not consciously colluding with her. Sometimes this can be difficult to believe, because it can be so easy for us to see what is happening; but were it not for my discussions with Zoe and the work I am doing with Lucinda, I doubt whether I would have been able to see the very subtle mechanisms which were in action below the surface. I find myself dependent on communication. Zoe and Lucinda trusted me enough to tell me what I needed to know to be of use to them, even when they were both hating me. One assumes that trust goes with love: sometimes it is a comfort to find that trust can also go with hate.

It is interesting to consider the problems I have described in other settings. Take for example the puddle experience (6). When Zoe found herself unable to forbid Lucinda to walk in the puddles because she liked to do this herself, Zoe did not in fact go in the puddles, but she *was* at that moment *Lucinda*, who was going in puddles.

Mothers of small babies also function in this special sort of way; they know how their babies feel, because they themselves are emotionally part of their babies. But there are mothers who continue to feel like this, so that their babies do not have the opportunity to become separate identities. There are also the mothers who are not able to be involved with their babies; they often attribute to their babies feelings which are really their own.

The capacity for what Winnicott calls 'primary maternal pre-occupation' is essential for people who are looking after babies on behalf of mothers. Students on the whole are likely to be able to be preoccupied with a baby, but may find it more difficult to be in sympathy with a toddler, especially if they are themselves a bit in need of mothering. Sometimes, by meeting their needs, it is possible to help them to meet the needs of others.

There is a term 'empathy' which I find very useful, and which means (I think) that it is one thing to get into someone else's shoes, but quite another to understand what it is like for the other person in his shoes, while remaining in one's own.

Zoe needed to be in with Lucinda (in the puddle), I needed to be in empathy with Zoe talking about her problems. Had Zoe been talking to me in general terms about work with children we might never have reached this point, but because we were talking about something real which had just happened and which still contained feeling, she could communicate and I could receive her communication.

When I spoke of students' needs and how these could be met, I was thinking especially about the possibility of a time and a place and a person ready to listen—even for only a few minutes—to communicate to about what has just been happening.

Zoe, in coming to understand the problems of Lucinda, also gained insight into her own and my own problems, and because of this we were able to work together more successfully.

I think that the use of a precise situation, such as Zoe's walk with Lucinda, could possibly be used for a basis of discussion with students working in residential nurseries.

9

The provision of primary experience in a therapeutic school, 1966

This paper is in a sense a summary of everything I had thought and written up to this point: it is also a statement about the Mulberry Bush school and the people who worked there during an important period. I found this a difficult paper to write (I read the communication in its original form to the Hampstead Child Therapy Clinic): several years passed before I could clarify and arrange the material for publication—I was too emotionally involved to find this an easy task. Had it not been for the skill and endurance of Mrs Elizabeth Irvine I am sure it would never have reached its final form: at which point the paper was published in the 'Journal of Child Psychology and Psychiatry'.

PRIMARY EXPERIENCE

Winnicott (1958) and others (Little, 1960; see also Chapter 2) have postulated a primary state of unity of the mother and her baby. In thinking about emotional deprivation I find it necessary to take as a starting point this state of unity at the very beginning of a baby's life. Freud (1926) wrote:

> For just as the mother originally satisfied all the needs of the foetus through her own body, so now, after its birth she continues to do so, though partly through other means. There is much more continuity between intra-uterine life and earliest infancy than the impressive caesura of the act of birth allows us to believe.[1]

In the course of normal development the separating out of

[1] This quotation also appears at the beginning of 'The residential treatment of "frozen" children'. It seemed more useful to repeat it in full, rather than to refer to the earlier paper.

mother and baby is a long and gradual process; at the completion of which the baby exists for the first time as a separate being and an integrated individual, absolutely dependent on the mother, but no longer emotionally part of her. If integration of the personality is to take place (usually by the end of the first year of life) the evolution of this process must not be interrupted. Interruption of this essential process, which mothers and babies work through together in their own time and in their own way, is in my view the trauma which lies at the root of the various types of cases of emotional deprivation referred to us (see Chapter 2).

The point at which traumatic interruption has taken place determines the nature of the survival mechanisms used by the child: the primitive nature of these mechanisms does not prevent them from being used in a highly complex manner. Winnicott (1963, p. 53) has said:

> All the rest of mental illness (other than psychoneurosis) belongs to the build-up of the personality in earliest childhood and in infancy, along with the environmental provision that fails or succeeds in its function of facilitating the maturational processes of the individual. In other words, mental illness that is not psychoneurosis has importance for the social worker because it concerns not so much the individual's organized defences as the individual's failure to attain the ego-strength or the personality integration that enables defences to form.

The emotionally deprived child is pre-neurotic, unable to experience guilt or anxiety, and functioning at various primitive stages of development. For a neurotic child there may have been inadequate continuity between the intra-uterine and postnatal phases, but nevertheless he has enough protective and protected environment to make it possible for him to build a separate personality structure, capable of integrating good and bad experiences and his responses to them rather than being helplessly buffeted by them. He is thus able, having reached integration because of 'good enough infant care' (Winnicott, 1958, p. 212), to embark on the long voyage of secondary experience. This is not true of the children under consideration here.

The children we select for treatment fall into several categories, depending on the stage at which interruption of primary experience took place.

'Frozen' children

The most primitive of these categories, that is to say the least integrated, is made up of those whom I have described elsewhere as the 'frozen' children (see Chapter 2); who have suffered interruption of primary experience at the point where they and their mothers would be commencing the separating out process, having been as it were broken off rather than separated out from their mothers. They have survived by perpetuating a pseudosymbiotic state; without boundaries to personality, merged with their environment, and unable to make any real object relationships or to feel the need for them.

Such a child must be provided with the actual emotional experiences of progression to separating out; thereby establishing identity, accepting boundaries, and finally reaching a state of dependence on the therapist. This kind of child cannot symbolize what he has never experienced or realized. (A 'frozen' child, on referral, will steal food from the larder because he wants food at that moment and for no other reason. The same child in the course of recovery may steal again from the larder, because his therapist is absent; this stealing will now be symbolic.)

'Archipelago' children

The next category consists of those who have achieved the first steps towards integration; so that one could describe them as made up of ego-islets which have never fused into a continent–a total person. For this reason we call them 'archipelago' children. These children give the impression of being quite mad whenever they are not being quite sane. They are either wildly aggressive, destructive, and out of touch in states of panic-rage or terror; or they are gentle, dependent, and concerned. They present a bewildering picture till one comes to know them and to understand the meaning of their behaviour. They too need to progress through the process of integration. However, these stormy children are not so difficult to help as are 'frozen' children, because the presence of ego-islets amid the chaos of unassimilated experience makes life more difficult for them. They are, from time to time, very unhappy and aware that they need help. The fact that some primary experiences have been contained and realized results in their having a limited capacity for symbolization, which facilitates communication of a symbolic kind which is not available to 'frozen' ones. Where 'frozen' and 'archipelago' children are concerned, treatment must involve the breakdown of pathological defences, containment of the total child, and the achievement of dependence on the therapist as a separate person. These two groups, in which integration has not been sufficient to establish a position from which to regress, are very different from those in the next category.

'False-selves'

Classifying the 'false-self' organizations, Winnicott (1960, pp. 142–3) writes:

> At one extreme: the false-self sets up as real and it is this that observers tend to think is the real person. In living relationships, work relationships, and friendships, however, the false-self begins to fail. In situations in which what is expected is a whole person the false-self has some essential lacking. At this extreme the true-self is hidden.

Having described other types of false-selves advancing towards health, he continues: 'Still further towards health: the false-self is built on identifications (as for example that of the patient mentioned whose childhood environment and whose actual nannie gave much colour to the false-self organization).'

The latter organization he has described as the 'caretaker-self' (Winnicott, 1960). This elaborate defence takes various forms, and is often difficult to recognize, especially because the 'little self' part of the child is carefully concealed by the caretaker (for example there may be a delinquent 'caretaker' which steals without conflict, on behalf of the 'little-self').

The first two groups, that is to say, the 'frozen' and the 'archipelago' children, do not adapt to demands in the way characteristic of false-selves and caretaker-selves. This is one of the reasons why they prove unmanageable in most residential setting;

there is no real little-self to be protected, but there is an embryonic ego capable of evolvement in a containing environment. Both false-self and caretaker-self groups need to regress to the point where development originally came to a standstill, often reaching a state of psychic fusion with therapist, from which they can advance once more to a more adequate integration as whole people.

I think of all these children as pre-neurotic (only integrated people can contain personal guilt and anxiety). They employ a variety of survival techniques, such as I have already described, which one may perhaps distinguish from defence mechanisms because of their primitive nature. One factor seems common to all: the experience of interruption of an essential illusion (Winnicott, 1958, p. 237), namely the mother–baby unity of the immediate postnatal period, due to premature failure by their mothers or mother substitutes in adapting to their needs during the first year of life. With this failure of the containing environment, they have been driven to shoulder the load of their separateness before independence could be achieved. The point at which this disaster has befallen them will determine the means of survival at their disposal.

Such failure can come about in many ways: for example, one mother may be unable to remain preoccupied with her baby for sufficiently long; another may be able to have an initial fused experience with her baby, but can only separate out by withdrawing concern; there may be actual separation of mother and baby, as described by many authors; or again, the father, who would have been the normal protector of the vulnerable unit, may have died or departed.

HANDLING OF THE CHILD

My thesis is that all these groups of children require the provision of primary experience which has, so far, been missing from their lives. There is no question of ego support at such a stage of treatment: the therapist, like the mother of an infant, must provide the total ego of organization until integration makes it possible for the child to establish his own ego.

The mother normally shares with the newborn baby an illusion that they are part of each other; this fragile illusion is protected by a 'barrier against stimuli' (Freud, 1922, p. 33) provided by the father and other helpful members of the household. What is real in this earliest phase is the perfect or near-perfect adaptation which the normal mother makes to her baby's needs. Disillusionment follows in the natural course of events, through the gradual failure in adaptation and consequent realization of separateness by both mother and child. All the children I have described have been exposed to some failure of this illusion at the outset of life, and therefore need to experience it, belatedly, before they can develop further.

Our task, then, is to provide such illusionary experience; by which I mean something felt in a here-and-now context which enables the child to make use of symbols in a way that he can fill in the gaps which have till now made continuity of experience impossible. We must provide this in a way which will feel real to ourselves and the children in our care; we can achieve this only by making perfect (although of necessity localized) adaptations to their individual needs. Perhaps this is akin to what Sechehaye (1951) describes as giving the psychotic child 'symbolic realization'.

The essential point is that one should be there to meet the child's indications of possible areas of adaptation, much as Winnicott (1960) describes the mother meeting the baby's spontaneous gesture. (It would be no use at all for us to think out and decide on an appropriate adaptation for a particular child.)

One day, for example, I was walking down the street with Marguerite. At the time I describe she was ten years old, and had come to us with an elaborate caretaker-self organization made necessary by early and traumatic separation from a very disturbed mother. Just at this moment she was emotionally exhausted and in the deepest part of a localized regression in which she was involved with me. I remember thinking, 'If she were really a baby, I'd pick her up and carry her home—as it is, what can I do?' As if in answer to my thoughts, Marguerite laid her hand in mine in a way that made it clear that in carrying her hand I would be carrying Marguerite herself. In this way she made it possible for me to provide the necessary experience.

It is essential in this kind of work that the therapist should support the child in such a way that the latter has a *complete experience*. This will not symbolize any previous experience, although it will be symbolized later, following realization. This experience must be felt as real, and worked through by child and therapist so that eventually the child is able to face and verbalize even the reality of his original deprivation, and to know that nothing can be done about this in objective reality. In order to achieve this, the pain and disillusionment must have been endured by both child and therapist; the former can only tolerate this in the context of a relationship based on complete experience. (The precise nature of such an experience depends on the individual emotional history and needs of each child.) I can illustrate incomplete experience in this sense by referring to that of an isolated child in a rage who eventually falls asleep from sheer exhaustion: the corresponding complete experience is that of a child who is supported through such a rage by his therapist, so that eventually he can be comforted and settled; he can go to sleep at last because he is ready to do so.

Perhaps one might say that in this sort of treatment 'the complete experience' may have to take the place of 'the correct interpretation'. It is impossible to interpret, because there cannot be symbols of a missing experience. This can be seen clearly in the connection of panic fears, panic rages, and panic despairs: the child needs help to go on to the end of the panic so that the experience can be completed.

The essential characteristic of panics which are so typical of these children is incompleteness—in much the same way that a nightmare is incomplete because the dreamer awakes from an unfinished dream. When the dreamer can complete the nightmare and then awake, it will become a bad dream; similarly, when the child in a panic completes the rage, terror, or despair and survives, the panic becomes a bad experience which can be contained, tolerated, and stated.

Babies imaginatively create their own mothers in terms of their individual needs (as described by Winnicott, 1958, p. 238). In the same way pre-neurotic children imaginatively create their own therapists. Both babies, and the emotionally ill children I am describing here, follow this creation by annihilation, and then create once more. Only if this process can be tolerated again and again can the next stage be reached, when the objectively real baby can find the objectively real mother.

I remember how individual were the needs of our own four babies. My own experience with each of them was also quite different; they have evolved into four very different people; and I know that subjectively they had, as babies, four different mothers. (Maybe they were also four different babies to begin with; there is much evidence of temperamental differences at birth.)

Vanno Weston, one of the teachers at the Mulberry Bush, had a nine-year-old girl called Pat in her group who expressed this very well. Pat said: 'At the home where I was before I came here, there were all of us children and the grown-ups who looked after us; here there is my group and *all the Vanno Westons!*'

There is nothing traumatic for the therapist to endure in the process of being 'created' by the child: on the contrary, this is a happy experience; obviously the risk of seduction and anti-therapeutic collusion is great in some cases. Very different is the experience of 'annihilation', which is so primitively destructive that one cannot talk about anything as personal as hate in this connection, and must be endured if treatment is to succeed. The child simply 'wipes out' the therapist; the therapist has to *feel* wiped out, rather than defend himself against the child. An interpretation in such a context becomes a defence, because it asserts the continued existence of the therapist. A common form of annihilation is for the child to cut off all communication with the therapist. For example, Robert, in this situation, said to me: 'I've had more than enough of you—I'm fed up with you', and did not come near me for a week. I did nothing about this, because I knew that he had wiped me out. When he returned, he re-created his illusionary me in a slightly different form, and we continued to work together.

Annihilation cannot be planned, any more than can creation, it must simply be endured as what it is felt to be, in terms of the involvement. Presently the child will re-create the therapist once more, because now he is ready to do so; but there will be pain every time annihilation takes place, which may be frequently. Once some degree of differentiation has been achieved there will be the gradual appearance of ambivalence, and now there can be real personal hate in the relationship. None of this can be organized, but providing one is prepared to go through this sort of experience with the child, the phenomena I have described will turn up in good time.

Much time and patience may be needed before a state of involvement can be reached. There are long periods when we must contain the child within the therapeutic environment of the school, waiting for the beginning of processes like those I have described. In the meantime, we do our best to ensure that those areas of personality which are functioning continue to do so. For example, the occasional child who has no learning problems should not lose ground educationally, although he may be a case of school phobia. He continues his education either through special teaching in a group, or if necessary, through individual tutorials. Marguerite (mentioned above) was able to keep her regression with me localized in this way, continuing her everyday life fairly normally; her education was seldom interrupted.

It will be remembered that caretaker-selves and false-selves need to regress before they can progress healthily, but that 'frozen' and 'archipelago' children must progress from the start. The first two groups have reached a point from which to regress, the second group must advance to integration, because they have remained either unintegrated or only partially integrated. The progression of an unintegrated child presents greater problems of management, because he does not feel in any way inadequate. He lives entirely in the present; there is no past to make him guilt-conscious, and no future to create anxiety. In the course of progressing to integration this kind of child finds himself unable to function in any field; having abandoned his delinquent survival techniques he feels utterly helpless, and goes through a phase of anaclitic dependence, during which he needs very special care.

John (aged ten years, a 'frozen' child who had reached this state) was dependent on Mildred Levius. He found her absence intolerable and talked about this to me, complaining of his feeling of emptiness. At this point it was possible for Mildred to establish adaptations as indicated by John; one of these was reliable supply of sugar lumps, another was a special sort of reading tutorial

combined with tea in the staff house. John was able to count on
this steady provision, and to replace desperate demands with hope-
ful expectations.

Lynn (aged seven years, a child in Mildred's group who seemed
to have a caretaker-self) had needed for some time a little walk
after her lesson group. During this walk, at intervals, she needed
Mildred to hold her upside down–virtually on her head. Now, at
a slightly later stage, she needed to be brought the whole way
round, so that the experience was completed with Lynn on her
feet again.

Robert (aged eleven years, a child with a caretaker-self)
acquired the nickname of 'Bedstead', and in my talks with him he
gradually allowed me to meet his little-self, which I suggested
could be called 'Cotstead'. The caretaker part of Robert, the Bedstead part, was severe and harsh: during one of our talks he was
able to explain to me that his ears and hands belonged to little
Cotstead–that Bedstead had no ears or hands. However, much as
we all tried to help Robert, he was unable to have the regression
which he so badly needed; until finally in Mildred's group Bedstead handed over the care of Cotstead to Mildred. Robert
managed this by building in his lesson group a model, which he
called his 'fourposter bed' (this was also Mildred). His hand could
be tucked up in the fourposter, and Mildred could look after him.
The savage Bedstead caretaker almost disappeared, and Mildred
took care of a very small Cotstead, who was at last able to begin
to learn (to be 'fed').

I have spoken of four groups: the 'frozen' ones, the 'archipelago' children, the caretaker-selves and the false-selves. I now
wish to discuss these groups and the various living-in treatment
approaches they need, in more detail.

Provision for 'frozen' children

For a 'frozen' child who has not integrated, the most important
experience to be provided will be the achievement of separateness
and the establishment of boundaries to his personality. This is a
slow and gradual emotional experience in normal development
(just as weaning needs to be slow and gradual); whereas in the
case of the 'frozen' child, separating out has been sudden and

traumatic. The 'frozen' child will have survived by preserving the illusion of unintegration, using merging instead of dependent leaning (see Chapter 2). Because such children have never arrived at the point of disillusionment and acceptance of separateness as individuals; they are perpetually struggling to remain fused with their environment, which, because they have not achieved integration, seems to them to be a normal state of being.

Interruption of mergers with adults or children produces suicidal panic. I have written at some length about 'frozen' children elsewhere (Chapter 2); here I only want to stress that we have to replace the illusion of being merged with someone else by the experience of finding – as it were – the boundaries of the self.

Peter (a charming, violent little boy of six years) tried for two hours to draw me into his panic rage, as a form of merger. I sat holding on to his hand, while he whirled about on his bed; biting, kicking and clawing me, and shrieking obscenities. This behaviour gradually gave way to isolated statements: 'I know I'll be dead by the end of this . . .' and 'Soon you'll be in a rage too . . .' and 'I know you'll be so scared you'll leave me in the middle, and I'll kill myself . . .'. I suggested that what he did not know was that he really existed, and had really been born; I also existed and had also been born; because of this we were both real people. I told him that I was not going to leave him to destroy himself; that it was safe to attack me and that I would not allow him to destroy me either; that I valued him; and that I would stay until he was through his terrible ordeal and out on the other side. (These comments I made sometimes in lulls, and sometimes at the top of the storm, when I had to shout to be heard.) Suddenly Peter asked: 'Like the other bank of the Thames?' I agreed that it was just like this.

We spoke about the Thames again a few minutes later, and I said that I thought that up to date he had been swept along by the current downstream towards the sea, but that I was asking him to swim across the current: that I knew how hard this was and what a struggle he was going through, but only by doing this was he going to find the other bank for himself, and prove to himself that it really existed.

I suppose that in classical analysis this would be regarded as reassurance made for the analyst's own benefit, but here was a statement of a primary experience which I made to the child because it needed to be verbalized.

At the end of a two-hour ebb and flow of panic rage, Peter was suddenly able to tell me – by now he was gasping for breath – that he was all right, would I wrap him up and feed him? He said, 'I am so thirsty.' I wrapped him in a blanket, in which he curled up exhausted but relaxed; I brought him a whole jug of warm milk, of which he drank every drop. I think that at this moment he established his body ego. Two months later he achieved dependence and a depressed mood.

Provision for 'archipelago' children

Provision of primary experience for what we call an 'archipelago' child is somewhat different, even though he must also progress to integration.

As I have already said, there are ego-islets which in normal development would gradually fuse into an established ego. In the case of an 'archipelago' child the break in development has taken place at the point where the baby was in the process of separating out, but where only some localized integration had taken place. The resulting 'archipelago' stage can give the appearance of disintegration, but in fact it is an early stage of integration and needs very special provision.

When we first knew Anthony he was on the one hand, the gentlest and kindest child, and on the other, the most destructive that I have ever met; the swing was from one moment to the next. Anthony's father had left home for ever when the mother–child unity still needed total support. Anthony said to me later in treatment, 'Poochie' (our little dog who had puppies at the time) 'is fed and looked after, so that she can look after her puppies. It would be awful if she had to leave them to go and get food for them – there needs to be someone to look after her *and* her puppies.'

Where Anthony was concerned, the whole team had to work together; each person making contact with whatever bit of Anthony could be reached at that particular moment in each context and by each person. My husband spent six hours sitting on the end of Anthony's bed one night because the child had asked: 'Will you stay till I go to sleep?' and he had answered 'Yes'.

Faith King took him to see the swan family on the River Wind-rush, and their talks together about the swans helped him to understand his own and his mother's problems. Vanno Weston gave him a purple sweet each morning. Joe Weston brought him an orange in bed each night. I had sessions with him 'on demand', which usually meant two or three times a week, when Anthony communicated with me in terms of a saga concerning a little mole lost in a labyrinth.

Between such episodes there was no continuity; Anthony would fly round the school attacking other children like a whirl-wind, throwing furniture about, smashing windows and scream-ing abuse at us—quite out of touch with reality. However, the ego-islets began to grow; a nucleus of ego was formed, the areas of havoc became gradually more limited, until within a year of his referral to us Anthony became a more or less integrated person.

I must add one more note about Anthony in connection with the purple sweet. Each child in his group had a special sweet each morning from Vanno Weston, whom her group called Vanno Sunshine because of her warm smile. Anthony's sweet, as I have already mentioned, was always a purple one. Richard, another child in the group, said one morning: 'I want a purple sweet!' Other members of the group said at once: 'Well, you can't have it because Anthony always has the purple one.' Richard sighed and settled for a pink sweet. Anthony was standing in the window through which the sunlight was pouring, holding up his purple sweet against the light. He had, however, noticed what had happened, and called to Richard, saying: 'Come and hold up your sweet and let the light come through it like I'm doing!' and when Richard did so Anthony said to him, 'All the sweets look the same when sunshine comes through them.'

This piece of communication not only showed us Anthony's use of symbolism, but also his newly found capacity for empathy.

Provision for false-self children

James, who came to us with an adapting façade of good manners, obedience and charm, behind which was tumult and confusion, had been through a period of regression with Faith King and was at the start of synthesis. One morning he asked Faith for a piece of buttered toast at the end of staff breakfast. Faith provided this at once, recognizing an appropriate form of adaptation which could be maintained without too much difficulty. James in fact continued to need his piece of buttered toast from his therapist for about eighteen months. Only Faith herself could make this adaptation, and reliability of provision was essential, this continuity having been absent in his babyhood. By the end of the eighteen months he no longer needed the adaptation, and at the end of three years he reached some degree of integration, albeit rather fragile.

Provision for caretaker children

Marguerite, describing her babyhood experiences, said: '. . . the wind blew, the bough broke, the cradle fell. . . . Why did the mother leave the baby in a cradle on a weak branch? Why didn't she notice the wind rising?' Indeed, she felt that it was only she herself who had taken care of the baby.

She was the first child with whom I attempted a localized regression within the Mulberry Bush. (I had brought children through total regressions in my private work, under very favourable conditions.) The journey down to the bottom of the regression, where the caretaker handed over to me and I was allowed to look after the very small baby–and the synthesis which followed, took about a year to achieve. My provision for her needs consisted of giving her a short session each day; in the course of which she slowly introduced me into her inner world. She described to me in detail a country at the bottom of the sea, where Jane Hook the pirate's daughter (the delinquent caretaker) and the shrimp (the little-self) lived with the Shaking-hand-fish (myself at the Mulberry Bush) and the Holding-hand-fish (myself alone with Marguerite) in a shell house built by the fishes and Jane Hook.

I had to gain the confidence of the caretaker part of Marguerite, so that I was allowed to help to take care of the little-self. At the bottom of the sea, the Holding-hand-fish and the Shaking-hand-fish helped to take care of the shrimp until the caretaker part of Marguerite was able to hand over to me altogether, and the newly integrated Marguerite became wholly dependent upon me for a time. She told me about this in terms of Jane Hook leaving the shell house and allowing the fishes to take over the shrimp.

I find that this kind of communication provides me with the means of making adaptations in a reliable way. I have to be very careful not to be tempted into making interpretations which would be irrelevant or even damaging because they were premature. As a fish I could say all sorts of things to the shrimp which as a person I could not yet say usefully to Marguerite, who was all the time realizing and symbolizing her experience in her own way.

I used no interpretation in the ordinary sense, at this stage, but really lived through this experience with her. Much later, when the shrimp had become completely dependent on the Holding-hands-fish, Marguerite used to trot behind me whenever I went to the Mulberry Bush, holding my hand, which I had to leave ready behind my back for her to take while doing all sorts of other things around the school. I also bathed her on Sunday evenings (this was when I always worked at the Mulberry Bush in some kind of practical way).

I was able to gain her very troubled parents' co-operation, without which treatment could not have been successful.

During the regression there was a disaster when I was away for a few days, and the shrimp shrank to a dot. There was another crisis when it fell into its bowl of porridge head first; no help could be obtained because the fishes had *not* installed a telephone. Annihilation came into the picture: Marguerite (in the Mulberry Bush) cut off all communication with me, and the shrimp announced that the fishes had gone for ever from the shell house and could never return. Of course from Marguerite's point of view she could really annihilate the fishes—one of the advantages of being prepared to work at the bottom of the sea! Later she recreated myself and the fishes with slight variations.

Eventually came the next great step, when Marguerite told me that the shrimp had grown too big for the shell house, the fishes and the porridge, and was leaving the bottom of the sea. The fishes helped to launch the shrimp, and Marguerite left the Mulberry Bush to go to a boarding school for less disturbed children.

On her last visit to the Mulberry Bush, Marguerite told me that the shrimp had just broken an antique jug which it had owned for years. I said that I felt the jug had served its turn, and could now be safely broken because it was no longer necessary. Later in the session Marguerite said suddenly, 'Why don't I feel you are special any more? Why, you are just Mrs D!' Disillusionment was complete, and I pointed out that now she was really Marguerite this meant that I could be really Mrs D. She replied with a little sigh, 'We will still know each other, but it will be different. . . . I suppose we will be friends!'

PROBLEMS FACED BY THE PROVIDERS

I want to say a little in conclusion about some of the difficulties faced by the treatment team—the providers.

When an adult becomes deeply involved with a child, both of them are naturally highly sensitive to the impingement of others on their relationship. We have evolved a plan for this stage of treatment which we call 'trio therapy'; in this the adult–child involvement is supported by a third person, whom we call the 'catalyst'. The function of this third person is something like that of the father in supporting the mother–baby unity. The provision of this support has proved an emotional economy, and has enabled treatment to proceed much more rapidly than has hitherto been possible. From the child's point of view, for example, when his own therapist is away the 'catalyst' will help him to tolerate this separation and to understand his own rage and misery in this situation. The therapist on the other hand, taking much-needed time off, is liable to feel rather the same as the mother who must at times leave her baby in the care of someone else. This 'mother substitute' must be known and trusted by the mother; in the same way, the 'catalyst' must be known and trusted by the therapist.

It will be realized that the therapist providing primary experience in a residential unit faces rather special difficulties. It is clear that any one worker can only go through this process with a limited number of children (in ten years I myself have helped twenty 'frozen' children to integrate). It is not possible to have more than two or three children going through the first phase of treatment at the same time.

The child will come to know the worker as he or she really is, rather than what the therapist hopes to be like. Such insight can be very painful, and is unavoidable in a context in which the child will be aware of so much—not only of the loved grown-up at his best, but also at his exhausted worst!

The therapist making this provision must face the fact that what can be provided is not only illusionary, but also inadequate, because the experience has to be localized, and because the relationship will inevitably be disturbed by the behaviour of other people. Above all, there is the fact that the therapist, however devoted, is not the child's own mother. The therapist will also be having an illusionary experience; in an involvement with a child such an experience—so like that of a mother with a baby—can seem very real. It is true that the therapist will have insight, and the support of the 'catalyst', but there is no 'barrier against stimuli' like that provided by the protection of the father and the home. On the other hand, the therapist will not be hampered by the load of guilt and anxiety felt by the mother of a disturbed child.

The particular emotional problems faced by the therapist who is thus involved with a child are, however, presumably to some extent the problems which would turn up if he or she were actually a parent. For instance, the integrated child may not grow up, as the therapist would hope, into a normal person making satisfactory identifications. The therapist's adaptations cannot be ideal and there will be limits to his capacity for involvement. For the child there are the early years of emotional deprivation and traumatic experience, and there will be many external factors likely to intrude into a treatment setting which makes use of the total environment. This is a difficult and painful realization, because of the amount of love and care which the therapist has given to the child.

The 'catalyst' supporter plays an important role in helping the therapist to tolerate these painful insights, even being prepared when necessary to impinge into the involvement, when separating out is unduly prolonged, and there is a danger of involvement turning into collusion; just as the father in a family would impinge into the mother–baby unity if he felt that it was becoming too much of a good thing. On the other hand the 'catalyst' will be in a position to support the therapist; for example, in assuring him that the current failure in adaptation is not in fact a final catastrophe for the child, that failing is not 'letting down'.

Usually it is a sound plan for the parents to take over the child at the stage where integration having been established, secondary experience comes into the picture. Often parents who have been unable to make adequate primary provision can successfully meet these later needs; the child may well transfer the image of the 'good therapist' on to the parents. We hear of this from parents and children subsequently, which is of course interesting information to receive; we also have the opportunity in some cases of watching a similar development at the Mulberry Bush, especially in deprived children whom we dare not risk sending into a new environment, however favourable, during such a critical period. The usual practice is for the deprived child to move gradually into another group. The relationship established with the new therapist will be secondary experience, a transference largely based on the primary experience with the first therapist; just as in analysis the transference to the analyst will be fundamentally based on the original experience with the actual parents. This move presents emotional problems for the first therapist; it is no easy task to hand over, however gradually, the child with whom there has been a deep involvement, but final separating out is essential for recovery.

Through my weekly individual and group discussions with the team, I have found that certain insights which we have gained together have been of value at these difficult moments.

A devoted mother, I have said, gives her baby a splendid start in life, but there are likely to be areas in which she may be inadequate because of her own personal difficulties; we are likely to fail for the same reasons. She must comfort herself with the thought that her husband, members of her family, friends, teachers and others will make up for her inadequacies. We, as providers, must console ourselves with the same reflection, and be able to let the child make good use of our failures.

A fear which has often surfaced in discussion is that the primary experience provided by the first therapist will be given away by the child to someone else. This fear is not well-founded, because it will not be the good complete illusionary experiences which will be transformed; these will be incorporated, they will really be part of the child by this time. Understanding of this makes the transfer of the child to another group more tolerable for the first therapist.

We should be glad, I suggest, if the child can find what we have not been able to give him with someone else at the Mulberry Bush, at home, or in a clinic later on; it is because of our emotional inadequacies that the child is needing compensating experience, just as the little child starting school (for example) may often find with his first teacher experiences which will compensate him for shortcomings at home.

Finally, it would seem to me that in any unit containing pre-neurotic children with a treatment team there will be providers, consumers (the children) and supporters (a provider in one situation at one moment may be a consumer or a supporter in another context). The balance struck at any time between provision, consumption and support will determine psychic equilibrium within the unit, and consequently the extent to which primary experience will be available to the children in treatment.

SUMMARY

The need for the provision of primary experience in the course of residential treatment of certain deeply deprived children has been considered in the context of therapeutic work in a boarding school for maladjusted children. The nature of primary experience, and means of providing this have been discussed. A distinction has been made between the needs of such children before and after integration as individuals. Some of the special problems faced by the therapeutic providers of primary experience have been noted.

Context profiles

An attempt to report on the progress of children
in a therapeutic school (1967)

This is a description of the beginning of a recent project, which in fact continues at present. We are, at the moment, engaged in building a form of reporting based on the idea of the Context Profiles, but more condensed and convenient. I read this paper to the Association of Child Psychology and Child Psychiatry, where members of the current team – Roger Stansfield and Dennis Branner – were also present and able to make valuable contributions to an interesting discussion.

The work of the team on this project seemed to me to indicate a new growing point in the school.

Mrs Barrett, our school secretary, was responsible for all the hard work involved in arranging the 'Profiles'. Because of her concern and insight she has prepared many papers and reports for us over the years, and we all owe her much gratitude.

The project I shall be describing has been carried out by the headmaster and the staff of the Mulberry Bush, working with myself as Therapeutic Adviser, over a period of four school terms.

There has usually existed a weekly staff discussion group of some kind in the Mulberry Bush (as in most therapeutic schools) during the past seventeen years; the nature of this discussion group has to some extent reflected the chequered history of the school. In 1960 Elizabeth Brown and I both reported to the Association of Psychiatric Social Workers on a staff group which she led for some time in the Mulberry Bush and which was of great value to us all. There were other periods when the team was too exhausted or under too much stress to face further evening work (at that time all meetings took place in the evening). Again, following reorganization of the school in 1962–3 and my own increased commitments in others fields, staff groups became more structured for various reasons and especially because of considerable changes of personnel, so that with many newcomers to be considered the discussions became seminars, out of necessity.

My own role, from this point onwards working for only two days each week in the school instead of full time, naturally altered: I found myself facing many of the problems of the outsider coming into a residential place (one of the problems which Miss Brown and I had considered in our papers). At first, I used the hour set aside for my weekly discussion with the team as an opportunity to explain something about my work with individual children (I selected the material with some care). I hoped that this approach might bridge a considerable gap between the team and myself: this gap was created partly because at that time it was administratively convenient for me to meet children in a staff house a little distance from the school, and partly because this was in the main a new team finding difficulties in accepting the kind of outlook which I seemed to them to represent and which they felt belonged to the past rather than to the present. I thought that by describing my own work I would be inviting criticism and questions, but this hope was not fulfilled. At other times we would discuss an article we had read, or a specific subject, but at no point did I feel that we had succeeded in establishing real communication. Working wholetime in the school I had been able to talk about children with grown-ups in context rather than in retrospect; now I was finding myself relatively out of touch with both staff and children (except for the few children who were in therapy with me).

Gradually it became clear that I could be of more use to the team and the children by having individual talks with the team members: once this plan was adopted, the discussion group began to be of value because people became more accustomed to talking about their work, alone with me. I began to wish that something could be found which was as explicit and definite as a therapeutic session, to provide a containing field for communication concerning residential therapy.

It must have been at this point that I started to wonder about 'the situation' in residential treatment as being comparable to 'the session' in psychotherapy. I thought that such a 'situation' needed to involve experience between the reporting adult and a child or children; an experience felt, realized, and communicable to others. Observations could not, in my view, be properly classified as 'situations' in this special sense, because observations have an effect on situations. One cannot, for example, observe a worker bathing a child; one can only observe an *observed* worker bathing an *observed* child: the very presence of the observer inevitably alters the situation. I realized that much of the reporting from the people in the school came under the heading of observation, rather than experience. It was unusual for the grown-up to discuss his or her feelings, either in the group or in the individual talks; on the contrary, the aim seemed to be to achieve what was felt to be professional objectivity – thereby avoiding personal involvement. It is in fact impossible to provide primary experience for emotionally deprived children without experiencing personal involvement: this needs, however, to be conscious and always for therapeutic purposes, rather than delinquent collusion.

Towards the end of 1964 there was another considerable change of staff. John Armstrong (the present headmaster) and Roger Stansfield (who became deputy-headmaster), who both came at that time, talked over with me the difficult problem of running the weekly discussion group in such circumstances. We concluded that – initially at all events – we should discuss material from outside the school. I made use of Winnicott's BBC talks concerning mothers and babies (1957), which seemed an appropriate basis for a group which had not yet integrated: consideration of the integration of the individual could help us to integrate as a group; the recordings made it possible for me to become part of the listening group. The way in which we work at the Mulberry Bush is largely based on Winnicott's outlook, so that this material was especially appropriate; it enabled the group to see how much in common there is between the experience of the ordinary devoted mother and the provider of experience for emotionally deprived children.

We continued to meet in the evening (at about nine o'clock): sometimes the meeting had to be cancelled, and usually two or three members of the group were away on leave, or too exhausted to come. At other times, members were still settling troubled children for the night, and occasionally I could not come myself. There was, therefore, a lack of reliability and continuity, which tended to keep discussion at a superficial level: this made me feel frustrated and irritable, which of course made matters worse, especially as the group was not sufficiently established for all this to be surfaced to a conscious level. John Armstrong and I talked about the current difficulties facing the group, and John suggested that we should transfer the meeting from Tuesday evening (nine o'clock till ten o'clock) to Friday lunch-time (one o'clock till two o'clock). Needless to say, we were at once facing a new set of problems, but these did not prove insurmountable, so that the group now had a continuous and evolving life, without any real breakdown. It is the work of this lunch-time group which I am going to discuss, although the Context Profile project actually started at the close of the difficult period of evening discussions.

I have already mentioned that I was beginning to think of 'the situation' as comparable to 'the session'. By now, I felt that the situation must be held in a context of time, place, and person. I hoped that eventually the context of the situation might become also the structure of the situation itself: but that, for a start, a week could represent the main time context, the school the place, and one child the person considered by the whole group. Time and place contexts within the main scheme (the week for a child in the school) could then be subdivided into more specific contexts within twenty-four hours of school life: i.e. getting-up time, meal times, lesson groups, 'inbetween' times, and bedtime. I asked the group to make notes on their own personal experiences with one child within one framework of context. I explained that by experience within a situation, I meant a happening between the grown-up and the child in relation to one another; not something observed by the grown-up which happened between the child and someone else. I mentioned at the outset that I would like to write something eventually about what we were trying to do: this was agreed upon by the team, and we embarked on the project.

At the first meeting I explained that when we had collected all these various experiences between grown-ups and children in the course of a week I would, with the help of our secretary, Connie Barrett (to whom we are much indebted), arrange the experiences in terms of the specific contexts. Thus all experiences reported in connection with getting-up time would be grouped together, and so on through the contexts, until bedtime. The whole report would cover a week (which was stated), but would be arranged as though covering a day. It was clear that the contexts would not be constant (no two meal-times would be identical). I felt, however, that the contexts were sufficiently exact in terms of time, place, and people to offset this disadvantage. Besides, as there were going to be many such profiles, there would be opportunity for considering the effect of variation of context on the situation.

It will be understood that this kind of reporting was not intended primarily as a description of the child (although there would of course be plenty of interesting material available in the profiles for use in reports from the school to clinics and local education authorities). I was much more concerned with a revue of a total situation in the place. We agreed that no experiences could be included in the profile other than those belonging to the particular week, although reference could be made, in the course of discussion, to previous experiences.

As I have already said, I asked the team to keep notes, which they could bring to the group: these notes could be arranged afterwards in terms of context. I thought that there would be ample time for discussion following individual communications; it seemed unlikely that all members of the group (usually about ten people) would have experiences to report in connection with one particular child in one week.

I knew that the group ranged from the people with a vast store of insight, knowledge, and experience to the novice students encountering emotionally deprived children for the first time. Students come to us from various courses, and from several countries, for periods varying from a week to a year. I knew that there would be comings and goings of visiting students, and possibly changes among the experienced staff: there would also be what I shall call 'newcomers' to the team, who whilst knowledgeable and experienced with children would be unlikely to have worked already with emotionally deprived children. I hoped that the context structure would help to hold this group together.

Just after we had started this project, an interested supervising psychiatrist suggested that perhaps we could produce profiles on six children, to be repeated over two further terms. The material which I shall be quoting in this paper has been drawn from these profiles (eighteen profiles in all, concerning six children over three terms).

In order to have an experience myself, I decided—with the approval of the team—to arrange one therapeutic session with the child under consideration, during the week: this became another experience available for discussion, and helped to establish my position as a member of the group.

I continued to have opportunity each week for individual talks with each member of the team, and John Armstrong, Roger Stansfield, Faith King and myself could all recommend reading to newcomers and students. It was therefore possible to assume some understanding in newcomers of the nature of the work in the school. Key people, especially John, Roger and Faith, were supporting and teaching newcomers and students at all times of the day and night! From the beginning, John made himself responsible for protecting the group and ensuring that we were able to work comparatively undisturbed, because he was looking after the children (it was at an 'inbetween' time for them, in any case). This meant that he was not able to contribute as much to the profiles as he would otherwise have done; on the other hand, he gave the group a feeling of security which would not otherwise have been available.

I had certain specific aims secondary to the primary task of pooling experiences:

1. I hoped that the possibility of accepting roles within functions (i.e. avoiding situations where a collusive or untenable role is accepted within another worker's function) would become clearer.
2. A principle of supplementing roles seemed to me of great importance. There could be the main provider of primary experience in a child's life; other workers could supplement this provision, thereby bridging gaps in the inner resources of the main provider and in his or her actual absence from the school. This way of working needs insight on the part of the person who is supplementing and also on the part of the person who needs to be supplemented.
3. I wished the newcomers to become aware of the contrast in experience between one worker and another in relation to the same child. Here, I hoped that splitting mechanisms would become apparent.
4. The members of the group would be sharing memories of experiences in this particular week; I myself would have something in common with each of them (individual discussions)

and would be contributing personal experience (the session with the child). I hoped that these facts would strengthen the group and also my relationship with the team.

5. I thought that the child care part of the team would find here an opportunity of linking their vital work more closely with that of the teachers.

6. Collusion is one of the many pitfalls in residential work. I was concerned that all the team should become aware of the dangers implicit in becoming 'good' in contrast to 'bad' other people in the child's life in the place; and of the same dangers in the team groups.

7. Adaptation to individual needs in a group is an essential therapeutic skill in providing primary experience, and one which often seems impossible to achieve. I hoped that the material provided by the key people would help the newcomers and students to see how this could be done, and how regression can be organized and localized.

8. I thought that newcomers in particular might become more aware of the implications of working as a member of a therapeutic team, especially when they themselves might not be the main providers and could easily resent the children's dependence on someone other than themselves. For instance: A, trying to comfort a child whose 'special person' B was on leave, might say, 'But you know B must have time off, now cheer up', instead perhaps saying to the child, 'You must be feeling awful with B away, I'm so sorry—I know how much you need him.'

9. I hoped too that discussion of experiences together might help members of the team to achieve empathy; to be able to imagine what it would be like to be in a child's shoes, while remaining in their own, rather than through projective identification to feel as though they had become the child through unconscious merger with him.

10. Emotionally deprived children must exploit because they cannot trust; they must make use of people because they cannot be dependent upon them. Provision of primary experience can lead to expectations replacing demands, but in the meantime exploitation is inevitable. I felt that awareness of tolerated exploitation for a therapeutic purpose might be com-

pared with the situation of being unconsciously manipulated (especially by 'frozen' children who seduce in order to exploit).

11. I thought that symbolic communication could to some extent compensate for the lack of direct interpretation, and that reflection (Axline's technique) could be safely and appropriately used also.

12. It was important that reassurance should be avoided at all costs; children should be allowed to be depressed—this could emerge in the material.

13. Because the traumata in these children's lives happened so early, the anxiety had been unthinkable; it could only be remembered through feeling. Panic is one way of remembering, and newcomers needed to understand the nature and management of panic, and the provision of containment.

14. Since the team would be constantly providing children with illusionary experience, there was likely to be an idealization: of the school, of the team, of their particular group or child, and consequently of themselves. Discussion of the profiles could make idealization apparent.

15. People in residential work often fear to lose intuition through gaining insight. I hoped that this fear would become less hampering through the informing of their intuition in a suitable emotional climate.

16. It is especially difficult for young workers to tolerate hate and rage in the children and in themselves. This might become more tolerable through finding that other people could stand being reliable hate objects, and that annihilation can be followed by re-creation.

17. I hoped very much that we would all become more easily able to allow children to make use of our failures in adaptation, and to learn to distinguish between failing and 'letting down' children in our care (as described by Winnicott, 1958, p. 312) in our attempts to meet their needs.

18. Since the experiences selected by the group would tend to reflect their own feelings about the children and each other at that particular moment, I thought that the pooling of projections could, without becoming a conscious process, nevertheless have an interpretative function (as described by Irvine, 1959).

At the time when we started to work on Context Profiles, the group consisted of:

John, *headmaster*
Roger, *deputy-headmaster*
Dennis, *teacher*
Faith, *teacher*
George, *teacher*
Margaret, *matron*
Karen, *deputy matron*
Donald, *child care worker*
Ann, *student*

Since it is a tradition to use Christian names in the school, I shall do so here.

A plan for the selection of children for profiles had also evolved. John suggested that we should choose six new children, to be profiled in the order of their arrival dates in the school. This seemed a practical basis for choice. Had we selected children who had been with us for some time, there would have been key members of the team who would know very much more about such children than newcomers. As it was we all started from the beginning of the child's life in the school.

Our first context profile was of Peter, during the week running from Wednesday 5 May, to Tuesday 11 May 1965. At this time the group was still meeting in the evening.

I shall quote this profile in full.

Name: PETER

Notes on particular context. Peter was suffering from a boil on the back of his neck during this week, which gave him a lot of pain and disturbed his sleep.

He had been moved this term from Faith's group to Roger's (the 'Bigs'), having had some primary experience with Faith. The reasons for his move were that Peter was tending to come to Roger's group and seek contact with him. The arrival of two new children in Faith's group made moves necessary, and this seemed the right step for Peter; initially he spent half the time with Faith and half with Roger. However, he came back quite frequently to Faith's group, and had plenty of contact with Faith.

A list of happenings follows, arranged in terms of times of day. Workers quoted in this list are John, myself, Roger, Faith, Donald, Ann and Karen.

Getting-up time. No unusual behaviour noted by anybody except Donald, who reported that Peter sometimes takes a long time to dress. A student who often works at the Mulberry Bush had told a member of the team during the previous term that Peter was wearing large thick socks which had to be tucked in round his toes; he claimed they had belonged to his dead father.

Meal times. Donald and Roger said that Peter's behaviour at meal times was found to be normal in terms of his having newly arrived from Faith's (the 'Smalls') dining room. He tended, as the Smalls do, to check up and protest if not satisfied, getting up from his place and coming to the serving table to do this. This behaviour was more exaggerated when Roger (in whose group he now worked) was supervising the meal.

Inbetween times (before and after meals, before and after lesson groups, etc., i.e. unstructured periods). John, George, Faith and Peter were in the office. George was not well and was going home to bed, when he complained, jokingly, about having no one to snuggle up to in bed. Peter said, 'Haven't you got a Teddy?' and he offered his own Teddy to George. George showed his appreciation, but refused the offer, whereupon Peter continued, 'Well, my mum has a Teddy she goes to bed with as big as you.' Faith explained that Peter's Teddy bear was a yellow one which belonged to her but was very much valued by Peter.

On another occasion Peter passed the office window carrying a very large Teddy bear, which in fact belonged to a small girl. He said to Karen, 'Look at my Teddy bear!' but it was quite clear to Karen that it was the little yellow Teddy bear that he really felt to be his own and which he wanted. Donald reported that he had helped Peter to make a chair and a cushion for this yellow Teddy bear.

John was in the office when Peter came in with his soldier's cap on the wrong way round. John felt that this was a recent development and that, indeed, wearing the hat was also recent although Peter had brought it with him from home when he first came. At that time he had looked after it with great care and had told John of the importance of its being preserved. It seemed likely that this actually was his dead father's soldier's cap, which was given to him by his aunt after his father's death.

John described Peter's bravery when John dressed the boil which had been giving him so much trouble. Peter was in great pain and could have struggled and protested. In fact, tears were flowing down his cheeks but he was absolutely co-operative and allowed John to treat the boil.

There was general agreement that contacts with Peter were only made where one happened to run into him in connection with some particular episode. He was not a child who came to look for just anybody, but was highly selective; his special contacts were John, Faith and Roger. He would only respond to an approach if he chose to do so. Karen remarked that she rarely met him alone; he was nearly always in the company of another child.

There were many comments about his being an 'outsider'. At this point in the discussion group a photograph was circulated which was of Peter when he was small, with his family . . . head hanging, looking depressed and unhappy and very much an outsider. Donald remarked that he was the only boy in his dormitory who was not a Cub.

Faith told of an outburst with Peter, in which he rushed away in a desperate state. This culminated in his telling her of his memory of a row which he had when he was out with his mother (he was probably referring to his aunt); he had felt that he wanted to run out into the street and get killed. This memory was very real to him, and was associated with his present state.

Peter's soldier's cap was for some time worn by another boy, Dougie. However, when Peter showed it to Ann or Karen, although it was in Dougie's locker, there was no doubt that it belonged to Peter and that it was very important to him.

Group time. Peter threatened to strangle Roger with his tie if Roger did not give him a sweet. Roger said, 'If you do that I will not be able to give you sweets.' Peter asked, 'Why not?', to which Roger replied, 'Because I would be dead.'

Peter wrote a story about a little creature on the moon. He (the little creature) saw a cow for the first time and was very frightened, hiding behind a locked door.

Peter's painting had always been remarkable. Roger mentioned that he thought it derivative, in that Peter took ideas from pictures in books; he did not copy these but used them as a basis for his work. Roger did not feel that his paintings reflected his inner life. (I think Faith disagreed with this in terms of her experience.) Earlier in the day Roger had described to me how Peter had asked him to help him with his writing by doing some writing for Peter to write over.

Peter returned to Faith for a cooking group. Faith had found herself afraid to upset him but felt that this was a wrong attitude at this point, so had refused to correct a mistake she had made in not giving him the right thing for his cooking. He demanded this and Faith refused, feeling this was an important change for her to feel it was right to do this.

Faith said that while in her group Peter was very group minded, although he was extremely difficult and demanding: while outside he only played with younger children. It was very important for him to be read to by Faith, but he only wanted stories suitable for small children.

Roger described him as a difficult person to have in his group; it was clear that one of the reasons for this was the recent move from Faith to Roger, with all its implications for Peter in terms of his own history.

Donald told the group that during woodwork group Peter made many boats. Just recently he made a submarine: he needed to make sure that it could sink and that the periscope would work, which he associated with breathing. It seemed that he enjoyed bathing here, in contrast with his fears of bathing at home.

Bedtime. Peter wanted Roger to try on the soldier's cap. Roger said that it was Peter's cap. Peter insisted so Roger put on the cap, whereupon Peter said that it did not look right on him (he could not turn Roger into his own father).

Ann mentioned giving aspirin to him when he could not sleep because of the pain from the boil before it burst. Peter called her one night after the boil had burst, and asked for aspirin, saying that he could not sleep unless she gave it to him, She refused, saying that she thought now he would find that he could sleep; there was in fact no further difficulty about this.

Ann said that another child in Peter's dormitory had wrapped up his Teddy bear, and Peter held up his own Teddy bear to show that it was also wrapped up.

While we were having this group meeting, Peter came down to the office, and Ann took him back upstairs. When she returned, she reported that Peter was very worried about Nicky (an asthmatic child) who was choking and retching: other children in the room had been frightening themselves with talk about ghosts. Peter appeared really concerned about Nicky.

My session with Peter. I had planned to have a session with Peter, as it seemed to be the best way of making a contribution to this report. I had a brief 'ice-breaking' session with him on the previous Friday. He accused me of not having talks with him; we discussed the problem of the time factor. I made a reference to the first time we met, and he developed this theme. He said that he would like to come and see me again.

When I went to look for him on the Tuesday morning, he refused absolutely to come; he was frightened of me, I think, and afraid of what might emerge in talks with me. His story about the little creature on the moon and the cow confirms this. He hid behind a door.

Discussion. There was considerable discussion during the collection of these happenings; the following points are just a few of those that came up.

The difficulty of knowing what was really going on inside someone as well defended as Peter gives importance to apparently minor details, especially when there is a possibility of symbolic statement or action which may give clues to the nature of his inner world.

The soldier's cap and the large thick socks, both of which Peter said belonged to his dead father and were inherited by himself, could be important in this way (in relation to Roger).

The move from Faith to Roger might be a premature one; it seemed, however, that Roger was being seen by Peter as a father who could take some of the responsibility off Peter's shoulders.

He might have further localized regression with Faith, or with Roger, or with both.

Peter probably had feelings of great fear of having to follow in his father's footsteps and be killed; if he was to follow father exactly he must *be* like father.

No one at home spoke of his mother. Perhaps, through stories (for example, the story of a voyage) he might begin to talk about the experiences at a pre-verbal level during his first year of life which can only be preserved in symbolic terms (he would not, I was sure, be able to talk about his later memories of his mother, at home).

The story of the little creature on the moon and the cow could refer to his meeting with me, and his fear of what he might discover if he gained insight (and also what I might find out about him).

Notes by me. The Teddy bear might be a transitional object, as someone suggested. However, I did not believe that this was so; but rather, that the bear symbolized a split-off part of himself which he could not yet let us know about, except in this symbolic way. The bear's needs might give us clues as to Peter's own regressive needs. In discussion of the profile nobody spoke of the Teddy bear as large as George, which Peter described his mother as having in bed with her. I felt that it would not be appropriate at the first meeting to bring this material forward myself: I followed the lead of the group in considering all the Teddy bear experiences which people had had during the week, and also the vicissitudes of the soldier's cap. The group was able to realize how apparently small and insignificant facts could, when brought together, give real clues to Peter's problems.

The boil and its treatment might have had symbolic significance for him; this could turn up later in pictures or stories (that is, when realization of experience was followed by symbolization).

My own impression was that there would need to be considerably more regression if this child was to achieve integration. There would be a problem here for Faith and Roger, because Peter would inevitably see them as his real parents, one of whom deserted him, and the other was killed. There must, however, have been some primary experience for a degree of integration to have taken place. Roger and Faith worked closely together to help him become aware of the inevitable splitting which had to take place.

It would be very important to meet his fantasies about his birth and his earliest experiences with his mother; he might be holding himself responsible for what happened to his parents. There would, of course, be his conscious memories of his father and mother; they were probably merged with his fantasies.

It would be easy to mistake Peter's acceptance of a delusional role (that of his dead father) with the normal process of identification, which would have to be reached eventually.

Further notes. I thought that Peter's acting out in the role assigned him by his aunt helped the team to realize how easily they could act out in terms of roles assigned to them by children or by other members of the team. The need for continuity of experience with Faith was obvious in the material, and the unavoidable interruption was seen as a danger. Although much of what was reported was more observation than experience, the team could see clearly the number of 'bits' of Peter to which they needed to respond, and how varied must be his needs. For example, Faith's failure in adaptation during the cooking period (following her provision of primary experience), in contrast to Roger's provision (the writing for Peter to write over). Roger was now the main provider.

Both in group discussion and later individually, I talked with the team about the difference between empathy and projective identification (in connection with Peter's apparent concern for Nicky).

We were troubled by the stoicism displayed by Peter, and felt that when he became more integrated he would be able to be much more unhappy; because in order to contain emotions it is necessary to have been contained oneself.

There was little evidence of adaptation to his special needs, because Peter had not indicated these yet, and had no expectations—only demands. However, the aspirin episode suggested that he was feeling his way towards adaptation.

No notes had been written by the team for this first profile: I thought that the group probably felt that it was for me to collect and arrange these valuable communications. I accordingly made brief notes at the time which I rewrote more fully at home after the meeting; I returned my notes to the team for checking, before they were typewritten and arranged. I found this a most tantalizing task; it was difficult for me to consider the material and make notes at the same time. In fact–because they wanted more time for discussion–the group gradually started to keep notes from which I could work. Eventually they decided to collect all material beforehand, so that this could be ready for the group meeting, thus leaving more time for discussion. I think that this spontaneous development was of great importance, and I was glad that I had not insisted on notes in the first place.

I had not evolved any clear idea as to my role. It seemed essential that the group should understand how much I valued their work: perhaps by carefully reporting their communications, and by helping Connie to arrange these to make a Context Profile, I would be showing my appreciation of their skills both as individuals and as a team.

Before they started to keep notes themselves, there was often no time for discussion or for me to read my own notes on my experience with the child. On these occasions I added my own work and notes to the profile after the meeting, and it was then available to the team.

Gradually we found it possible to consider experiences in the course of presentation. Insight, therapeutic skills and experience varied so much from person to person that I found it necessary to select points for comment with great care; I made many mistakes. However, with the experienced members of the team (the key people) this was not a consideration, except in so far as material could be too disturbing to newcomers. My impression was nevertheless that less experienced workers could tolerate description and discussion of key people's experiences, and could sometimes gain insight through such audience participation. Something of the same kind is described by Miller (1966), when group leaders discussed their work with each other in the presence of the group.

The eighteen profiles were at last completed, leaving me in considerable doubt as to the value of such an approach. The team themselves asked for a discussion the following week on 'reporting'. This was a very interesting meeting. A member of the team (who tended to idealize his group) spoke of his feeling that there was a 'halo' round his reporting. A student (I think) said that there needed to be two kinds of reporting—one for heaven and one for hell. In general, the group thought that there might indeed be two kinds of reporting; one for those who understand our special work, and one for those who do not. Someone said that if she reported as she really *felt* about happenings, what she stated would certainly be misunderstood by outsiders. Another person thought that it would be impossible to write 'inside' reports for outsiders, because one could not write enough. It was pointed out that bits and pieces out of context would be worse than useless. However, there was a place for such 'inside' reporting within the school, which could be made available to outsiders in touch with our work.

At one point I said that it was perhaps natural that we should want to present the children and ourselves as 'good' to other people; it was quite difficult to describe both the children and ourselves as we really are (I was reminded of mothers of small children out to tea with relations or friends). I suggested that we might report single experiences from now on; not necessarily for other people, but for ourselves—the group: I suggested that we could talk in this 'inside' way among ourselves without a 'halo'.

We decided that the best plan would be for each member of the group to bring 'an experience' to the meeting; these would be briefly reported and the group would choose which happening should be discussed by us all.

The first experience reported was by a comparative newcomer, who described clearly and movingly the brief loss of his own boundaries in a merger with a child who was in a state of panic rage. The worker had not acted out in any way, but knew that for an instant he was without identity. He now felt secure enough to communicate this happening to the group. The group responded in a concerned and undefended way, knowing very well how terrible it can be to be caught up in another person's panic, however briefly.

So far we have needed to consider each experience; I think that gradually the group may choose one happening which has importance for all of us at that moment in terms of the school's emotional life.

Lastly, a few words about the group itself. A residential team has much in common with the Eskimos, as described to me by Professor Franz Fromm. Until recently (when civilization brought inevitable changes) it seems that the Eskimos never fought among themselves; there was no delinquency. This people was united against the common enemy—the cold—against which they waged an unceasing war. A residential team, especially in a therapeutic school, is always at risk from outside pressures of one kind or another. There will, at the same time, be protective and supportive agencies also outside the school. People providing primary experience, however, are inevitably highly vulnerable and sensitive, which causes them to draw closely together in a persecuted way against possible impingement. Such a group tends to be suspicious of outsiders, and this is, I think, understandable.

In relation to the treatment team, I started as an outsider, and to some extent have remained one; only I think not as threatening as at first. When my work in the school is finished I go away and do not return for several days: the team remains in the situation and cannot withdraw. This is a just cause for resentment which is often felt. There were many occasions when I became acutely aware of current crises within the group, often between members of the team; obviously I heard about all kinds of difficulties in the school during individual weekly talks with John and his staff. I found it important to remember that if I broke through the solidarity of the group by interpreting such tensions, I would be leaving breaks in much-needed defences (the integration of the group being precarious). Interpersonal crises in the life of a therapeutic school are constantly arising; the pattern varies from moment to moment. Outside pressures (management, economy, social attitudes, and so on) can instantly affect the emotional climate of the whole place in a positive or a negative way. I know that Caplan (1959) has found 'crisis' a suitable state in which to effect changes in attitude. My own work has been an attempt to prove with the team that the primary task can continue to be carried out, regardless of crisis. After all, mothers went on being preoccupied with their babies during the Blitz.

There were moments when I thought that the project would break down. For example: at one point members of the team complained that, because the group now met at lunch-time, there was no longer a main meal on Fridays (a sandwich lunch was provided which we ate while we talked). Quite a lot of tension ensued before an arrangement could be made by John for an early solid meal. I simply said how glad I was that such a plan had proved to be possible: interpretive comment could have caused havoc. Now and then the profiles were interrupted by a group request for a discussion on some special subject: here again, I did not interpret, but merely accepted the need for such an interruption.

Miller (1966), writing about the use of small groups in staff training in the penal system, states: 'Thus psychologically un-trained staff are constantly exposed to the psychological stress of being in interpersonal situations with highly disturbed human beings.' The presence of key people in the group gave constant support to the newcomers and students who were reacting to this stress.

John, Roger, Faith, Dennis and myself were able to speak of failures, and the use made of failure by children. We were also able to talk about our own feelings, and to speculate how much such feelings could affect the situation. I hoped that the newcomers and students could identify with our toleration of inadequacy and doubt.

Play as therapy in child care, 1967

I read this paper last summer (1967) to a child care course at the North-western Polytechnic. This was in itself a rewarding experience, and has been followed by a series of seminars during which I have been able to discuss the paper with members of my audience, in terms of their own experience.

I think that a definition can usefully be made between spontaneous play, therapeutic play groups, and play therapy: and that therapeutic play groups could make a valuable contribution to residential child care in homes, schools and hostels.

I

Lili E. Peller (1955), in a paper entitled 'Libidinal development as reflected in play', classifies the main features of children's play characteristic of successive stages of normal emotional development. She describes:

1. Narcissistic play—the child with himself.
2. Pre-oedipal—the child with his mother.
3. Oedipal—the child with both parents.
4. Post-oedipal—the child with others.

Writing of narcissistic play, she says:

> In the earliest months the playing infant appears interested in the parts of his body; in their functions and their products. Gratifications and their counterparts—deprivations—stay in the immediate neighbourhood of body needs ... remember that gratifications as well as frustrations are not yet accompanied by words or symbols.

Peller goes on to consider the child's play at the stages listed above, and summarizes as follows (the examples are my own):

1. Narcissistic play which is purely idiomatic; for example, a baby

playing with his toes, or with his mother's body as part of his own.

2. Pre-oedipal play, which can encompass another as an object; for example, a baby playing peek-a-boo with his mother.
3. Oedipal play which can be shared by several subjects and where theme and contact are communicable; for example, a toddler playing house with his parents.
4. Post-oedipal play, which takes forms that are predicated on step-by-step communication and mutual understanding; for example, a game of hide-and-seek with other children, according to agreed rules.

Peller does not, however, speak of 'integration' in her description (the essential process which must have taken place between stages 1 and 2); nor does she describe 'transitional experience' (Winnicott, 1958), in the course of which babies start to make use of symbols to bridge the gap between themselves and their mothers, as they separate out from a primary unity with their mothers to become individuals in their own right. I wish, therefore, to add 'transitional play' to Peller's classification, and to make a clear distinction between pre-integrated and post-integrated play. It would not, I think, be helpful to try to fit the phases of play to particular age groups. You are aware that integration as an individual normally takes place towards the end of the first year of life; however, in the course of residential work with deprived children of any age, workers will observe play belonging to all the phases described here. Peller's statement, that babies in the first phases are unable to think in words or to make use of symbols, is very important to us because there are many deprived children who are still limited in this way; their needs for play are very different from those of integrated children, who can symbolize. After all, words are symbols, as are the letters which form them.

We cannot assume integration in deprived and disturbed children, and it is this fact which creates tremendous problems in all aspects of management, including play. The baby at the beginning is contained by his environment; his mother (supplemented by others) is the environment which contains him. He is not yet in a position to contain experience; he is only able to reach such a position through the primary provision made by his mother's adaptation to his needs (described by Winnicott) so that he has eventually enough experience with which to build a self. The self is made of experience, and it is only on a basis of enough experience that he can become a *container*. He is then able to contain further secondary experience, because he can realize and symbolize what happens to him. He is no longer at the mercy of 'unthinkable anxiety' (Winnicott) which can only be remembered by feeling: panic is a good example of such memory by feeling. Symbolic play becomes an important field in which to sort out his experiences— to 'cope' with them; verbal communication links him with other people, so that he can describe what he is feeling to himself and others.

Many of the children technically described as 'deprived' are nevertheless integrated, having had a good enough start to their lives. They need plenty of facilities for play, and can make good use of these. The play of these children comes into the later categories. You will remember that Peller says 'their play can be shared by several subjects; theme and content are communicable' and 'they may use play forms which are predicated on step-by-step communication and mutual understanding'. Integrated children can play in groups; they enjoy games with accepted rules, such as ball games, hide-and-seek, or 'grandmother's footsteps'. They play 'house' or 'hospital', they paint, model, or build, and this play enables them to find relief from conflicts and tensions, which they can express and resolve in symbolic terms.

In residential places, however, one would expect to find other children who are emotionally as well as technically deprived; who have not had sufficient primary experiences to build selves, who are not containers, but need themselves to be contained if they are ever to achieve integration as individuals. They are unable to make use of play forms which would seem appropriate to their age and intelligence (the later phases of play described by Peller): on the contrary, they are likely to disrupt such play. Far from using games and toys—a dolls' house, draughts, or paints, for example— these emotionally deprived children will be more likely to destroy the toys, smear the paints over themselves and other children, break the furniture in the dolls' house, and generally wreck the situation for everybody, making it impossible for other more integrated children to make use of play provision in a meaningful

and valuable way, and causing 'play disruption' through impingement.

I suggest, therefore, that in residential places we should think
of two main types of play group; one for integrated, and the other
for unintegrated children. Both the play material and the type of
adult support provided for these groups should be firmly based on
the degree of individual integration: on the capacity to contain
(the integrated) and on the need to be contained (the unintegrated).
Of course integrated children can have areas of non-ego functioning, just as unintegrated children may have limited fields of ego
functioning. Nevertheless, there will be an overall picture which
can make such assessment feasible, and in any case the grouping
can be flexible.

We could say that where there is ego functioning there must be
opportunities to function, but where there is no ego functioning there
must be *provision of containment*. This applies to all fields of management, but here I am thinking especially about play. The children
whom we are containing may well need the first kind of play
described by Peller. She speaks of this, you will remember, as
being idiomatic, i.e. special to the individual concerned. She
remarks that there are neither words nor symbols involved at this
stage. She talks of narcissism, i.e. the play does not relate to others;
the mother is included only as part of the child.

We are thinking also of transitional play, because unlike Peller,
we need to be especially concerned with a more detailed consideration of phases of play which belong to the era of pre-integration.
Transitional play is part of transitional experience, to which I have
already referred; the essential bridging to the increasing space
between the mother and the baby, which is a normal and tolerable
process, without which there can only be a traumatic break leading
to a state of deprivation.

Provision of play for unintegrated children must include idiomatic and transitional opportunities (later we shall be considering
what this means in practice). Provision for integrated children
will need to be made in a way that acknowledges the ability of such
children (2) 'to encompass another as an object', (3) 'share with
several subjects . . .', and (4) 'make use of forms of play based on
communication and mutual understanding'.

Bearing these phases in mind, we now have some sort of a

framework, within which to consider the use of play in a residential place. I shall be thinking about children whose ages range from roughly three to twelve years; however, many of the principles involved apply also to play with adolescents.

II

I assume that in any group of children in a place there will be representatives of various stages of evolvement, on the journey to more-or-less integration as individuals, and that facilities for such various types of play need to be available at one time or another. How can such provision best be made? One grown-up can play with one child with comparative ease, at whatever stage of integration the child may be at that moment; nor will the grown-up have too much difficulty in running a play group of children who are functioning at the same sort of level, whatever that may be: the difficulties appear when there is conflict amongst the needs of a group of children who are functioning at various levels. Perhaps one could call this play-incompatibility. I am sure that you have all had to deal with this fundamental problem; it has much to do with integration, with the establishment of identity, and with the recognition of the identity of others.

Let us assume that there are sixteen children in a residential place, and that there are, let us say, two people available to play with these children for an hour after tea. Sixteen children can also be seen as two groups of eight: the selection of these two groups could be worked out by the people of the place. In fact, I think there would need to be a sort of assessment discussion, within which the people caring for the children could pool resources of observation and experience in order to decide the point of integration reached by each child. The two groups could then be planned on a basis of such an assessment; one group would be for the less integrated children–the ones who need to be contained.

Factors which could be used in this assessment:

1. The capacity to play with others without disruption.
2. The ability to communicate, especially in a symbolic way.
3. Respect for others and awareness of other people's needs.
4. Capacity for tolerating envy in respect of other people's gifts and achievements.

5. A lack of the need for total attention—the need to be the *only* one, different from the others (either as protegé or as scapegoat.

I think that on this basis one can make quite a reliable assessment of suitability for an integrated or an unintegrated group.

So here we are with two groups of selected children, one group of integrated, one group of not integrated children: we have suggested a time (an hour after tea), and we have the leaders of the groups—two people who might be looking after the children anyhow. But who are these people to be? I think there must be general agreement about this, whoever may be chosen for this particular kind of work. Certainly it would be a help if hierarchy could be forgotten, if the two people chosen could be simply those who found it easiest to play with children without feeling guilt (i.e. without feeling 'this is a waste of time' or 'children can play on their own', and so on). The decision must rest with *the person who is running the place*, who accepts great responsibility and whose decisions must be justified to supervising and inspecting agencies. When, therefore, there is a junior and less experienced worker who for one reason or another has developed such an idea—a play group for example—he or she will need to bring it to the head of the place (be it a school or a home) for consideration. It would be worse than useless—in fact, actually destructive—for a play group to be launched split off from the life of the place. We have learnt that there is no *one* person, alone, who can help deprived children; only someone *supported by other people* can do this kind of work. It follows from this that there must be a lot of discussion and planning before play groups can be launched as an integral part of the life of the place.

The play groups could take place in a garage, or a workshop, or the living room, or even in the play room. If the two groups must run in parallel, between five and six o'clock in the evening, perhaps—then there will have to be two places for play at the same time. Ideally the play group place should not be in use all the time; a living room presents snags. There could be a cellar. I suppose there is a great deal of variety, but if the worst came to the worst, perhaps a play hut could be built—a simple prefabricated building with a wall radiator and an electric light. If there really is only one place available for such special use, this should be reserved for the unintegrated group, for reasons which will become apparent as we proceed.

Now we come to the problem of equipment.

Provision of material for integrated children. The integrated group could make use of glove puppets, which are easy to make from papier maché and scraps of material. They will need paints (powder paints), sugar paper or newspaper, large brushes, and mugs for water. They may like to use masks, which can be made from papier maché. There could be a dolls' house with furniture and a family of dolls. A sand tray and water could be important; a couple of small screens could be used in all sorts of ways—as a house, a shop, or a hospital. Then there could be games; draughts, ludo, and cards, for example. Clay is better than plasticine. I am sure that the children's teachers could help with planning and make suggestions, especially in regard to where to buy cheaply and well.

Provision of material for unintegrated children. The second group (made up, as you will remember, of children who need containment and who are functioning at a much earlier stage of development) will need rather more special provision. They can make use of large boxes, big enough to contain a child. Other ideas which could be helpful are: blankets, cushions, etc., for nesting material; soft toys (teddy bears, and so on); feeding bottles filled with orange juice; a mirror; materials necessary for finger painting; a large jar of sweets of various colours; glove puppets; story books suitable for reading aloud; sand and water; and equipment for blowing soap bubbles.

You will see that there is some degree of overlap between the two lists. You may find it advisable to alter these lists; flexibility is essential in all arrangements for play groups. I only wish to indicate some kind of frame of reference within which to start two play groups in a residential place.

The room, shed or garage in which the unintegrated group will play will need to be as uncluttered as possible. Children who need to be contained need a reliable environment, geared to their needs (just as they need continued and reliable care), so that the arrangement of equipment, once decided, should be constant. A large cupboard in which toys, etc., can safely be stowed away between play sessions would be better than shelves, especially if both groups will be using the same room.

The integrated children *could* play in a living room; however, there are difficulties involved. You will find it hard to alter the room sufficiently for the children to feel that this is a different and special place, and that you in this context become a different and special person.

I am now imagining the possibility of these two play groups making use of a special play room, perhaps on alternate evenings. These play periods would not be directed: suitable materials and equipment such as I have described would be available and within the reach of hand and eye. The grown-up would not be concerned with 'good behaviour' during these times; 'good manners' would not be relevant. The worker would, in this setting, be a therapist; his or her role in regard to the play group would be different from that at any other time in the twenty-four hours. The worker and the children would be sharing a very special kind of experience during these brief periods.

People working in residential places sometimes tell me that they have very little time to play with the children in their care. There are many practical tasks to be fitted into the day: physical care, administration, maintenance, cooking, mending, and so on. Often they say to me, 'If only there was just a short time when one could just play with the children.' Listening to them, I get the impression that 'playing with the children' is regarded as a luxury which they cannot afford—an 'extra' rather than an essential factor. I am quite sure that a planned play group, at a given time in a given place, would not only be valuable, but could even be essential. Furthermore, I think that the feelings released in the play group and also in the leader of the play group, whilst sometimes disturbing, could nevertheless relieve tensions in the life of the place. This can only be the case, however, if the grown-up is prepared to accept the responsibility of being a therapist. Such a play group is therapeutic; and for this stage of affairs to come about, certain conditions need to be fulfilled.

Axline (1947) describes total acceptance of the child. She says:

Complete acceptance of the child is shown by the therapist's attitude. She maintains a calm, steady, friendly relationship with the child. She is careful never to show any impatience. She guards against any criticism and reproof—either direct or implied. She avoids praise for actions or words. All this calls for vigilance on her part. There are innumerable traps into which the unwary therapist might fall. The child is a very sensitive being and is apt to catch the most veiled rejection of himself on the part of the therapist.

This, for you, working in a residential place, means that although a few minutes earlier you were scolding Michael for making such a mess, or urging Janet to get on with her homework, now in this setting you (*the same person*) are accepting Michael and Janet as they are at that particular moment in that place; not needing to *direct* them in any way (except in regard to safety). You may feel that such a change of role must be disturbing to the children, and that at the end of such a period of undirected play Michael and Janet could tend to be disrespectful, disobedient, and so on. In fact, such a reaction is likely to turn up at first, but presently the children will sort out the roles for themselves—that is to say, you as a child care worker and you as a therapist. I work in this way myself with our private patients who live in our house, with an age range of from nine to seventeen years. Most of the time I am a grown-up managing a group of children: I am often critical of their behaviour—I get cross, I refuse to put up with this or that. However, for one hour in most days I am a therapist, and they talk with me alone and make use of me in a very special way, which is deeply different from any other time.

In the residential school for maladjusted children where I work as a consultant, the teachers find that at one time they can be critical—authority figures—while at another they can be running non-directive groups, in which their comments are for the most part attempts to reflect what the child is feeling. It is true that one is not treated with what people term 'respect' in this context, but on the other hand one is trusted in a rather special way; one may even be allowed to enter the inner world of the child whom one may have 'known'—without knowing—for a long period. Communication at such times becomes either symbolic or pre-verbal (the child may only communicate through *actions*). A small boy in the therapeutic school said recently to his teacher, Liz Greenway, 'I hate when people are just opening their mouths and noises are coming out but they are not really *saying* anything.' Often what we say to children, and they say to us, becomes stereotyped; in a play group communication can come alive.

Axline lays down eight basic principles for non-directive play therapy. I think that these principles are relevant to the special kind of playing with children which I am discussing here, and later I shall quote them in full. You will observe that the grown-up attitude which she describes would not be appropriate in some fields of the child's life. If a child says suddenly, 'I don't want to go to school today', we cannot help very much by saying, 'You feel you don't want to go to school today', because we and the child usually know that he *is* going to school this morning, and that he can accept this fact. In the same way he can say that he doesn't want to go to bed, or wash his hands before tea; we can understand that he does not want to do these things, but we can usually rightly insist just the same, and he can tolerate our insistance. However, if in a play group a child says, 'I want to smash that dragon' (a puppet), we do not need to say, in this special setting, 'But that would be naughty'; we can just settle for 'You feel you want to smash that dragon.' (Perhaps this boy's name is George? This is the sort of thing to keep in mind.)

I am now going to consider Axline's eight principles, and discuss how they apply to residential therapeutic play.

1. 'The therapist must develop a warm, friendly relationship with the child, in which good rapport is established as soon as possible.'

Here, the fact that our 'customers' are already known to us may make the establishment of such rapport unnecessary because it has long since been achieved. However, the children will also have assigned us specific and personal roles in their lives, so that initially there may be difficulty in accepting us in this different climate. Perhaps an important point to bear in mind would be, that in this special context, anything which has happened during that week or day becomes irrelevant.

2. 'The therapist accepts the child exactly as he is.'

I have already spoken about Axline's concept of total acceptance of the child. If we can just accept the child in *this* place, at *this* time, as he or she *is*, we may escape the temptation of relating the way in which the child behaves in the play group to his behaviour in other contexts. Total acceptance could mean that when Johnny wants *everything* in the play group we do not say, 'There you go, Johnny, grabbing everything as usual', but we might say instead, 'Johnny feels he must have everything—it must be awful for him to feel like this.'

3. 'The therapist establishes a feeling of permissiveness in the relationship, so that the child feels free to express his feelings completely.'

Johnny, at breakfast, must say 'Please' and 'Thank you' and be polite to others. At school, too, he must be respectful to his teacher, and this is as it should be. However, in the play group, if Johnny is to feel free to express his feelings and to be totally accepted—for an hour—then he may be rather rude to you, but he may also show you that he loves you. You will see a better and a worse Johnny than you would meet in other contexts. If he is free to say what he likes he will probably not *do* anything antisocial; freedom of speech can serve as a valuable safety valve.

4. 'The therapist is alert to recognize the feelings the child is expressing and reflects these back to him in such a manner that he gains insight into his behaviour.'

This kind of awareness is difficult to achieve; it depends on how much insight we have gained ourselves and how much we understand our own feelings. The more of this self-awareness we have gained, the more we can understand the children in our care.

Possibly, just because we are playing with Johnny and the others, just because we are not teaching, training, nursing, or supervising, we may be free to wonder more about the meaning of the play: for example, when a very quiet, good child becomes a savage giant when he is wearing a mask, we may wonder what hate and helpless rage may be seething inside him from behind the calm exterior he presents to the world. So that when the giant roars and rages you may find yourself saying, 'This giant is very angry about something—I wonder what made him so angry?' and perhaps the child talking as the giant may tell you important things about himself, about his *inside* reality.

5. 'The therapist maintains a deep respect for the child's ability to

solve his own problems if given an opportunity to do so. The responsibility to make choices and to institute change is the child's.'

For example, we can respect the giant's feelings; we can indicate such respect by the way in which we respond to the giant's rage. We can respond to what the child-as-a-giant says, making it clear that we can accept the giant's decisions *within the framework of the play*.

6. 'The therapist does not attempt to direct the child's actions or conversation in any manner. The child leads the way; the therapist follows.'

This, I think, confirms what I have said earlier. We are not teaching or training, we are doing therapeutic work.

7. 'The therapist does not attempt to hurry the therapy along. It is a gradual process and recognized as such by the therapist.'

Most of us think in terms of progress as improvement, recovery, and above all, change. Change there will be, but not if we are trying to *bring about* change in children rather than *support* them in evolving–changing–in their own special and individual way and in their own good time. We cannot hurry this sort of process: I think that the best plan is not to worry about change, but simply to continue to maintain a supportive reflecting role in relation to the child.

8. 'The therapist establishes only those limitations that are necessary to anchor the therapy to the world of reality and to make the child aware of his responsibility in the relationship.'

This principle for play therapy laid down by Axline brings us to the important question of limits. How permissive should we be? Where do we establish boundaries? I think that we must use sense and sensibility to determine limits in a play group. Much of Axline's work has been done with individual children; she acknowledges the difficulties inherent in group therapy of this kind. There are various views on the subject of 'limits', and I feel that the wisest plan is to set them as they are reached. For example, you would not allow children to hurt you or each other, to break windows, or to urinate in the sand tray. But it would be a mistake to announce a list of limits. Most groups will establish boundaries and remain within them.

These eight invaluable principles would seem applicable to

therapeutic play of the kind under consideration here. The principles apply to play with both integrated and unintegrated children, with the exception of the 'limit' problem (8).

As I have already said, unintegrated children need to be contained: they may actually need to be held. They are aggressive and destructive; we often have to supply the missing boundaries. Anticipation becomes especially important—awareness of impending play disruption and its interruption at a sufficiently early stage, to preserve the coherence of the group. One comes to recognize the first signs of such disruption and to localize the 'Storm Centre' (Redl).

We are now in a position to compare any group of children playing in the presence of an adult with the kind of group we are thinking about here, where the play group has a therapeutic purpose.

I think that it is especially the *attitude of the grown-up* which determines the nature of the group. Often someone who is supervising children's play will only intervene if necessary; in this situation the grown-up is not often involved with children, unless he or she is actually taking part in a game. The person who is running a therapeutic play group is deeply involved; contributing to the individuals and to the group as a whole; responding, reflecting, and sensitive to every mood and feeling.

The children in a spontaneous play situation may communicate with the supervising grown-up, and are likely to appeal for judgment in regard to 'fair play'.

Integrated children in a therapeutic play group will make use of the grown-up in a different way. More integrated children will draw the grown-up into their midst; asking for assistance, talking about their paintings, communicating with him or her from behind a mask, or with a glove puppet.

Unintegrated children will be seeking opportunities for regression: they will need to be fed, to be wrapped up, to be tucked into a nesting box, and to be read to (another way of being fed). They will indicate their needs, once they know that you will meet them whenever possible.

One must be prepared for surprises. Quiet children may become noisy and aggressive; noisy, tough children may turn into pathetic and trusting babies. Even the more-or-less integrated children may need to regress now and then; quite normal children regress in the course of an illness and become deeply dependent on the person who takes care of them. In an ordinary play group children do not tend to regress.

You may feel that there are many deprived children who do not need any kind of therapy, but only normal recreation. However, most children who are not living normal lives in their own homes have problems, however well they are coping with them; once in a while they need to find themselves in a situation where they can be absolutely themselves. The play group can often offer them such an opportunity, in a way which normal recreational activities cannot do.

The ordinary play time can take place in the garden, the living room, or the play room. The games that children play in the garden are different from those they play indoors. Children will play during any 'in between' time. A therapeutic play time needs structure; because what happens within the session is fluid and changing, the structure must be reliable. So a play group needs to happen in the same place, at the same time, and with the same person. This is true of all therapy.

III. HAPPENINGS

The happenings which follow have to do with various play groups with which I have been involved, at one time or another.

1. The first happening which I am going to describe took place on a wet winter afternoon, when, for various reasons, I had to play with twenty deeply disturbed children in one large room. We had no play equipment: there were tables, chairs, and mats on the floor, but little else. Because the group was so large and play material was lacking I suggested that we could play 'Desert Island'. Since the group seemed to accept this idea, I put one mat at the end of the room, and arranged all the furniture against the walls (the children by now were helping me) turning one table upside down on the floor. I explained that the mat was a desert island, the upturned table a ship, and the rest of the floor the sea. Before I could say any more, a crew had manned the boat, led by a very

determined captain–four children and a captain squeezed themselves aboard and prepared to set sail. All the other children sat with me on chairs and tables round the walls. We all waved as the ship set off on its long voyage. By now, the captain and the crew were eagerly discussing the treasure they hoped to find, and the dangers they would have to face. Suddenly the captain exclaimed, 'The wind is rising!' At once the children round the walls began to make the sound of a threatening storm; one boy banged a biscuit tin so that lightning flashed and thunder rolled all around us; the waves grew higher and higher until eventually the ship was wrecked and the sea was dotted with desperate sailors swimming for their lives. The captain and three members of his crew succeeded in reaching the desert island, but one sailor was drowned. (The audience by now *was* the storm; at the same time they shrieked to the crew to swim to safety on the island. They accepted the death of the sailor who was drowned as inevitable, saying, 'He didn't really want to live.')

Now the captain and his crew lived on the island for a *long* time (about five minutes, in reality); they built a hut, lit a fire, killed and cooked and ate wild animals, and caught fish (all this was talked about and mimed). Suddenly they saw a ship–should they leave the island? They were undecided, but the audience shouted: 'You want to go home, in the end.' So the captain and his crew were rescued by the passing ship and the audience cheered; the drowned sailor was pulled out of the sea and 'came alive again'.

During this adventure I perched on a table with some of the audience. I said very little except when someone involved me in the drama. There were calls for help from the captain, 'Are you going to let us drown?' I replied that he must feel that no one was helping them. The captain replied, 'We've got to do it ourselves!' One of the crew asked me, 'Shall I stay for ever on the island?' I said that it must be difficult to decide whether to go or to stay. One of the audience shouted: 'You've got to decide.' Presently, after a lot of discussion, a new crew set sail and there was another voyage, storm, and shipwreck on the island. Although the main structure was fairly constant, each voyage was highly individual.

The children all made use of this game in valuable ways. Certainly their lives had been stormy voyages; often there had been family shipwrecks: the island had something in common with the therapeutic school which they would one day leave. Here, in symbolic terms and without direction, they could safely act out some of their deep problems.

This group was made up of a mixture of integrated and un-integrated children. The integrated ones set the pace, made use of the symbols I offered them, and communicated at a symbolic level with the other children and myself. Unintegrated children were 'carried' by the group. The sailor who was drowned was not integrated and was overwhelmed by the force of the storm. My role was essentially a supporting and reflective one. I gave no advice, and there was no need for intervention.

The Desert Island game, as played by this mixed group, had elements belonging to most of the phases of play which I have listed earlier. For example, the drowned sailor was not really aware of the others; his play was idiomatic, in that he did not relate to the rest of the crew or to the audience—he 'drowned' for his own private reasons. The game was shared by several subjects; theme and content were communicable. All the integrated children made use of symbols (the storm, for example). At certain points the play suddenly settled between one child and myself (the child encompassing another as an object), for example, when the captain shouted to me: 'Are you going to let us drown?' There was not much evidence of form predicated on step-by-step communication and mutual understanding; the game developed spontaneously. Much of the game had a transitional character; the children were essentially bridging gaps. My particular choice of game and symbols had been intended to provide such an opportunity.

2. This happening concerned five very difficult and unmanageable children, in the same school. The group was indeed made up of those who were too disturbed to work in a lesson group—so they came to play with me. We met in a small room in which there were a table and several chairs; there was also a high, broad windowsill which turned out to be important. We had paints, paper, etc., some glove puppets, and some cushions and blankets. The five children were all resentful (feeling rejected by their own groups); none of them were integrated, and two were in fact psychotic.

David and Stuart started a slanging match full of obscenities; John charged round the little room making a loud roaring sound;

Peter wrapped himself up in a blanket and huddled in a corner; Tom climbed onto the windowsill and curled up on it in a foetal position. I sat and waited. Presently David and Stuart found the glove puppets; they put them on–one on each hand–so that presently there were four puppets arguing and threatening each other and me. I collected two puppets myself and tried to communicate with the children's puppets, but this broke down at once. David and Stuart threw away their puppets and started to wrangle again, and to prod Peter, who was still wrapped up in a blanket.

Tom (curled on the windowsill) suddenly woke up, and took a flying leap into the room, upsetting the paint water. All this time John had been charging round, still roaring steadily–the total sum of noise was ear-shattering. I said, rather loudly, that I wondered what fierce animal was roaring so loudly, and John paused long enough to inform me that he was of course a lion. Presently he allowed me to make a den out of chairs and a blanket; tucking himself into the den he reached tranquillity through containment: indeed he spent the rest of the session in and out of his den, with only occasional roars. I put a cushion under Peter's head and made an arrangement of blankets for Tom on the windowsill, in case he should return. By the end of the session, things were fairly calm, but there was no real group–just five isolates trying to find holes into which to crawl. At one point I held Stuart to prevent him from actually attacking David.

This was a group of unintegrated children: these five were far more difficult to manage than the twenty I have described previously. They made little use of symbols, although the lion became important to John in later sessions. There was no real contact with me through communication, my role was to reflect; but it was also to establish boundaries, to provide containment, and to hold if necessary. The play was narcissistic, except for the wrangling between David and Stuart; these children were not in touch with each other or with me, as separate people.

3. The third happening which I am going to discuss I have also described in another context elsewhere. It concerns a group of eight children: we were playing in the garden. The group decided that they wished to make little nests out of twigs and grass. They asked me if I would provide eggs to put in the nests. I

offered the possibility of small squares of chocolate, which they accepted. The children all made nests, with varying degrees of skill, and brought these to me to be filled (I should note here that I neither praised nor criticized the nests). I asked the first child, 'How many eggs?' and he replied, 'Four.' The second child wanted five eggs. The third child, Roy, wanted *one* egg. I just reflected what he said, giving him the one egg, and murmuring, 'Roy wants one egg.' I thought to myself that this child–who was very greedy and loved chocolate above all things–nevertheless needed so much to be *the only one* that this symbolic experience became more essential than the chance to eat several pieces of chocolate.

Here one can see a child making tremendous use of play, finding opportunities for symbolic experience which could *feel* real to him. The other children in the group had their own personal experiences; each nest was, in this sense, unique. In the course of this happening my role was essentially that of acceptance and support. The group–especially Roy–were having important and creative feelings: children who had reached despair were beginning to hope again. I asked no questions, because questioning could have been intrusive.

Here, I think the play was mainly transitional; the children were not really playing with each other, but they all included me in their play; the nest and the 'eggs needed contributions from the children and myself, building bridges between us. Although every child in the group decided to make a nest, their play remained pre-oedipal. Each child encompassed another as an object (myself). There was little connection between the children: for example, no one (except for my reflection) commented on the fact that Roy wanted only one egg; neither, for that matter, did they remark on the child who asked for five eggs. There were lifelines, of a sort, from each child to myself.

These happenings are not as relevant as they should be, for the purpose of this discussion, in that all the children described were deeply disturbed–basically emotionally deprived–at various stages of recovery in a therapeutic school. However, it so happens that my work had been with such children, and I have drawn on my own experience. Perhaps the acute nature of this kind of disturbance may highlight the points that I wish to make. In any case, there must be many group happenings in your own experience which you can subject to the same scrutiny.

What follows now is imaginary, although most of the material has turned up at one time or another. I am going to try to describe a fictional happening; seen first as an educational experience, then as a spontaneous supervised play period, and finally as a therapeutic play group. I feel that such distinctions are worth teasing out, because they tend to become confused.

I am choosing to describe a group of eight unintegrated children, their age range five to twelve years, playing with a child care worker whom they know fairly well.

1. *The educational play group.* The grown-up is in the room when the children arrive. She has taken a lot of trouble to arrange the play material on the tables and shelves. She asks each child what he or she would like to do, and provides material accordingly.

Three children say that they will paint—the paints are ready mixed. The grown-up gives each child a piece of paper and a brush, discussing with them what they will paint. One child is lying on the floor; the grown-up gently raises him to his feet, saying in friendly tones, 'Come along, Peter, this is play time, not bedtime!' The two remaining children wander about in a vague sort of way. The grown-up manages to collect them and settles them at a table on which stands the dolls' house. One of this pair hits the other, and the grown-up intervenes and begins to arrange the furniture in the dolls' house while the children sit silently watching her. Presently the grown-up looks at the pictures the children have painted, praising good efforts and making constructive criticisms.

2. *The supervised, spontaneous play group* (with the same children, adult, setting, and material). The grown-up and the children come in together. The grown-up has some mending with her. She settles near the window and starts to darn a sock. One child asks permission to get some water for painting; the grown-up gives permission, asking him at the same time not to make a mess. Another child comes and talks to the grown-up, perhaps about a television programme. Two of the children start playing with puppets. This begins as a sort of fairy-tale, but rapidly degenerates

into a battle, with the puppets being used as weapons. The grown-up takes the puppets away, saying that if they cannot use the toys properly they may not have them. The children sulk in silence. One child lies in a corner doing nothing; he looks as if he is dreaming. No one goes near him.

3. *The therapeutic play group.* The grown-up comes into the room with the children. She has already put away the dolls' house, but she has left blankets and cushions in corners and under tables, and also a couple of containers (a large tea-chest and a laundry basket). She sits on the floor in the middle of the room with a puppet on each hand. A child asks 'What shall we do?' and the puppets on the worker's hands discuss this, saying how difficult it is to decide what to play with. Different children argue with the puppets. Another child lies down on the floor, and the worker puts a cushion under his head and wraps him up in a blanket. The child says, 'I don't want to do anything,' and the worker replies: 'You don't want to do anything, perhaps you just need to *be*.'

By now there is nest-making in progress; children are fixing up safe places into which to tuck themselves. The worker helps where she feels needed: for example, a child in a tea-chest asks to be completely covered up and dark, and the worker makes a roof out of a blanket. Several children specify particular soft toys that they want to hold. One asks for a baby's bottle (already filled with orange juice) which the worker gives him. Suddenly there is a fight over a toy; the grown-up has noticed which child is the aggressor, and she holds him very firmly saying that she knows how angry he must be feeling. The attacking child is in a rage and screams. The grown-up goes on holding him, and the other children pay little attention. The child screams 'Leave me alone!' and the grown-up, understanding what the child may mean, says that he is afraid that she will leave him alone . . . he calms down.

I would like now to draw attention to the little boy lying on the floor in the course of each happening. You will have noticed that in the first case he is gently picked up and told, 'This is play time, not bedtime', and he adapts to the demands made of him; in the second happening he passes unnoticed because he is not presenting difficulties, he hibernates; in the third happening, his behaviour is seen as regressive. He is treated as someone in need of very early babyhood experience, and he responds to the adaptation made to his needs. He is now aware that not only is he being taken care of, but also that someone is caring about him—as he is at that moment and in that place.

SUMMARY

In this paper I have tried to catch the wind. Erikson has said (1950):

> Modern play therapy is based on the observation that a child made insecure by a secret hate against or fear of the natural protectors of his play in family and neighbourhood seems able to use the protective sanction of an understanding adult to regain some play peace. Grandmothers and favourite aunts may have played that role in the past; its professional elaboration of today is the play therapist. The most obvious condition is that the child has the toys and the adult for himself and that sibling rivalry, parental nagging, or any kind of sudden interruption does not disturb the unfolding of his play intentions, whatever they may be. For to 'play it out' is the most natural self-healing measure childhood affords.

I have tried to contrast integrated with unintegrated children and to compare their needs in the province of play. I have also attempted to clarify the therapist's role in a therapeutic play group, and to demonstrate the differences between this role, an educational role, and a supervisory role.

What I have been putting forward is the suggestion that child care workers, although not psychotherapists, can nevertheless do valuable therapeutic work of a special kind. I am suggesting that some of this already existing play could be channelled into non-directive play therapy.

I feel that there is a need for support for workers running such play groups, and that opportunity for discussion could be invaluable and perhaps essential—at first, anyhow. Perhaps some such opportunity could become available; in any case there could be discussion in the place about the happenings in the play groups: this would be valuable for the people in residential work who are trying to learn more about the children in their care.

Clare Winnicott (1963), talking to social workers, has said:

Of course we shall not always understand what is going on or what they are trying to convey to us, and often this does not matter. What matters most is that we respond in a way which conveys our *willingness to try* to understand. And it must be obvious that we really are trying all the time. This in itself can provide a therapeutic experience.

The children in a special play group will do and say things that we shall often not understand; but by reflective techniques and total acceptance we can help them to become more truly themselves. I believe that such work could be both practical and valuable.

Glossary

Anaclitic is a word used by Freud at a stage in his thinking, when he wished to state that the sex instincts 'lean up against the self-preservative instincts'. This term is sometimes used as a synonym for dependence, as if a child leaned up against a mother-figure; this is the sense in which I have used the term.

Archipelago is a word I use to describe a clinical state which indicates a state of fixed partial integration in a child's personality. Ego nuclei (Glover) have never fused or have become diffused. The consequence is that the personality is made up of functioning areas which are unrelated to the non-functioning areas where no integration has taken place.

Catalyst is a term borrowed from chemistry. A catalyst enables a chemical reaction to take place. A third person may facilitate a reaction or an interaction between the child who is the consumer and the person who is the provider in a primary experience.

Containment describes the provision needed by deprived children: that is to say, it describes a containing environment that aims at holding the child and the child's feelings.

Emotional deprivation is a term used to describe a failure of containment and its consequences. In some cases the containment was adequate and then failed, whereas in other cases there may have been an environmental failure from the start.

Frozen. I call a child 'frozen' who has early been broken off, rather than separated, from the mother. By the use of this term I intend to convey the idea of a child who has become well-defended against repetition of unbearable mental pain. The 'frozen' child, if untreated, is a candidate for delinquency.

Hibernation, a term well known in biology, can be used to describe a child's low level of existence maintained over a period of time. This is a kind of 'ticking over', and represents a form of childhood depression. Clinically this state is to be found among deprived children who are potentially but not actually antisocial at the time.

Merger. I use this to describe a symbiotic bond, where one person merges with another or a group in order to escape responsibility of identity.

Primary experience. I use this term to refer to experience belonging to the first year of life, without which integration as an individual is impossible. Primary experience may be given to the baby by the mother-figure, or may be offered at a later date by the therapist.

Reality annexe is a term I use in referring to a delinquent child's manipulation of someone preserved intact outside the immediate environment.

Symbiosis. A biological term whose use pretends to describe essential *emotional* interdependence. Clinically one needs to be prepared to find a pseudosymbiosis, in which what appears to be a primary unity is artificial, and therefore unreal and unproductive.

References

AICHHORN, A. (1935) *Wayward youth*, New York, Viking.

AXLINE, V. (1947) *Play therapy*, Boston, Houghton Mifflin.

BALBERNIE, R. (1966) *Residential work with children*, Oxford, Pergamon Press.

BETTELHEIM, B. (1950) *Love is not enough*, New York, Free Press.

CAPLAN, G. (1959) 'Mental health consultation', *Concepts of Mental health and consultation*, Children's Bureau Publication no. 373, U.S. Department of Health, Education and Welfare.

ERIKSON, E. (1950) *Childhood and society*, New York, W. W. Norton

FENICHEL, O. (1945) *Theory of neurosis*, New York, W. W. Norton.

FREUD, S. (1922) *Beyond the pleasure principle*, London, Hogarth Press.

— (1926) *Inhibitions, symptoms and anxiety*, Hogarth Press.

HARTMANN, H. (1954) 'Contribution to discussion of problems of infantile neurosis' *The Psychoanalytic Study of the Child*, vol. 9.

IRVINE, E. (1959) 'The use of small group discussions in the teaching of human relations and mental health', *British Journal of Psychiatric Social Work*, vol. 5, no. 1.

KLEIN, M. (1944) '*Emotional life and ego development of the infant, with special reference to the depressive position*', Controversial series of the London Psychoanalytic Society, IV.

LITTLE, M. (1960) 'On basic unity', *International Journal of Psycho-Analysis*, vol. 41.

MILLER, D. (1966) *Human relations*, vol. 19, no. 2.

PELLER, L. (1955) 'Libidinal development as reflected in play', *Psychoanalysis*, vol. 3.

REDL, F. and WINEMAN, D. (1951) *Children who hate*, Glencoe, Illinois, Free Press.

SECHEHAYE, M. (1951) *Symbolic realization*, Monograph series on Schizophrenia, New York, International University Press.

WINNICOTT, CLARE (1964) 'Casework and agency function', in *Child Care and Social Work*, Codicote Press.

—— (1963) 'Face to face with children', *New Thinking for Changing Needs*, Association of Social Workers, Dennison House, London.

References

WINNICOTT, D. W. (1957) 'The ordinary devoted mother', nine broad-cast talks; reprinted in *The Child and the Family*, London, Tavistock.

—— (1958) *Collected papers*, Tavistock, London.

—— (1960) *The maturational processes and the facilitating environment*, London, Hogarth Press.

—— (1963) 'The mentally ill in your caseload', *New Thinking for Changing Needs*. Association of Social Workers.

Index

Consultation in Child Care

Consultation in Child Care

Barbara Dockar-Drysdale

Foreword by Robert Tod
*Central Council for Education and Training
in Social Work*

To our children,
Sarah, William, Charles and Caroline

Contents

Foreword

If you are working closely with unhappy and angry children, or if you have responsibility for supporting and helping staff who are professionally involved with children, I believe that these papers will speak to your condition. Such work makes pressing demands on our personal resources, our caring and empathy, our insight and self-awareness. We need to draw upon our memories of childhood stress and apply what is valid from this to our own work with children. We need too the capacity to acknowledge the mutual dependence of members of staff on each other as well as the interdependence of staff and children. From time to time also it is important that we should make public what has hitherto been private and particular, and examine and test our practice and give our ideas to others in order to see if they are real and reliable.

This is the exercise on which Mrs Dockar-Drysdale has been engaged in the last few years, and as we read this second collection of papers, originally given as spoken addresses, she communicates to us the essential unity of her feeling and thinking. The papers are based on her experience of therapeutic work with children or consultancy with staff, which has been informed and deepened by her own study, reflection and analysis, clarified by theory and here expressed in a statement. In reading her chapters, we are drawn into accompanying her in the process of experience, realization and conceptualization.

I found that the papers said most to me when I read them in a reflective way, pausing from time to time to compare her insights with my own experience or to match, if I could, her clinical illustrations with situations I had encountered. I am sure that those readers who are involved with disturbed children in a residential setting will repeatedly find their own experience refocused or given significance by the discoveries made or clarification given by Mrs Dockar-Drysdale.

The present book carries further the experience and theoretical concepts presented and discussed in the author's first volume of papers, *Therapy in child care*. Readers will find that knowledge of the papers in the first book provides a necessary background to understanding these further papers. The present book is much more than a restatement of previous theories. In reading it I was constantly impressed by the way in which Mrs Dockar-Drysdale's thinking, founded on the work of others, has moved on and developed, so that here original concepts are presented in a new context for the first time.

At the risk of anticipating the contents of the book, I should like to mention those new concepts or insights which caught my imagination or confirmed my own experience: the classification of stress into simple stress uncomplicated by guilt which is bearable and complex stress which can be sometimes intolerable (ch. 1); the disabling effect upon staff of the force of unconscious envy (chs. 1 and 10); the need of visiting parents for a 'safe place' within the residential establishment, (ch. 2); the acceptance of there being no clear lines of demarcation between the therapist and the patient, the staff and the child, all needing supportive relationships to enable them to develop as human beings (ch. 5); the study and analysis of the needs of children rather than of their symptomatic behaviour provided in the two chapters on Need Assessment (chs. 8 and 9); and the description of the delusional equilibrium which is found in some establishments, where the overt task is frustrated by the existence of an anti-task that is outwardly denied (ch. 10).

Other readers will find other aspects that are valuable to them, perhaps the clinical case studies that are always vivid and apropos of the introduction to the theories of other writers, D.W. Winnicott, Klein or Sechehaye.

Mrs Dockar-Drysdale believes that in therapeutic work with children, unexamined intuitions are not enough; our work with disturbed children must be conscious, disciplined and professional.

In publishing her papers, she is sharing with us her conscious and disciplined presentation and examination of her professional experience and working concepts. I believe that many practitioners in residential work will find in this book the stimulus and encouragement that they need to develop their own thinking and practice.

Robert Tod

January 1973

Introduction

This second collection of papers records my further experiences and thoughts concerning the therapy needed by emotionally deprived children in residential places. These later papers will certainly be easier to read if the first collection *Therapy in Child Care* is already familiar, but chapter 5, 'Meeting children's emotional needs' should cover most of the essential ground for readers who are not used to the concepts involved.

Most of my earlier work was carried out within the Mulberry Bush School (a school for maladjusted children which my husband and I founded many years ago): it has only been during the last four years that I have become aware of just how great is the number of unintegrated children in residential care. I have been working now for some time as a consultant to the Cotswold Community for delinquent adolescent boys, and have also been involved during the same period with a wide field of work in child care. I have come to prefer running workshops to giving lectures, so that many of the papers in this book have been a basis for a day's work with my audience. I have also discovered that it is pleasant to be interrupted – that is to say, I often ask my audience these days to stop me at any point which they would care to discuss with me.

The death of Dr D.W. Winnicott has been for me, as for so many others, an irreparable loss. I hope I have incorporated enough of what he taught me to continue to make use of his work.

I am most grateful to the many people with whom I can talk over experiences and realizations. I would especially like to thank Richard Balbernie and John Armstrong for all the help they have given me. My secretary Kate Britton has once again with unfailing skill and care arranged and edited these papers. Without all this help the book would not have been completed. None of us can work alone – perhaps this is the theme of this second collection of papers.

B. Dockar-Drysdale

January 1973

I

Problems arising in the communication of stress

I read this paper at a refresher course run by the Association of Workers for Maladjusted Children, in 1968. I had been for some time rather out of touch with the Association so that it was pleasant and stimulating to be talking with this particular audience once more. The discussion which followed the paper revealed the evolvement which has taken place during the last ten years in the treatment of disturbed children. I found myself thinking of our early days, and of how, although there was a long journey ahead, at least we had made a start on the right road.

The newborn baby expresses stress as soon as any inner or outer disturbance upsets its psychic equilibrium: this is as true of excitement as it is of pain. There is no need for communication to be established between mother and baby, because for the mother the baby's cry comes from within herself; she hears and responds to its need as she would to her own. If this primary maternal preoccupation is lacking from the start, the baby is doomed to emotional disorder, unless a mother substitute can take over who is capable of this preoccupation and can establish a primary unity.

A mother responds without thinking to delicate variations in tone and quality to her child's cry; what action she takes will depend on what she feels about the particular cry. People working with disturbed children in a residential place need to be able to feel a child's stress at this primitive level. I have heard people working in the Mulberry Bush say, 'There's Jenny crying again, but she's alright', or 'Quickly, I must get to Jenny – there's something wrong'. To an outsider there is little variation in the quality of Jenny's cry, but for people who are closely in touch with this borderline psychotic child (who often cries) there are nuances in the quality of her crying which they can feel because of their sensitive preoccupation with Jenny. This is something more primitive than empathy.

As babies develop, integrate into individuals in their own right, and begin to communicate verbally, the picture changes to some extent. A toddler who is wailing can explain through his tears that his teddy has disappeared, or that he has a pain in his tummy; his mother can help him to search for teddy, or to ease his pain or help him to endure it. Sometimes, however, the basic stress is not being directly communicated: the momentary loss of teddy may have triggered off a much deeper fear of losing his mother; the 'tummy ache' may be in itself much less painful for him than an underlying dread of dangerous 'bad' feelings or intolerable excitement inside him. His mother will intuitively respond to this deeper level also.

Severe stress remains, as at the beginning of life *unthinkable*. Panic is an extreme example of unthinkable stress: someone in a panic cannot communicate what he is feeling; it is only after he has recovered from the panic that he can gradually and with help begin to describe this awful phenomenon. This is true of adults as well as children. One could say that stress remains or becomes tolerable if and when it is communicable. Many people – grown-ups and children alike – can communicate stress in retrospect; few can do so while actually in a *state of stress*. They react, of course – much deviant behaviour is in an indirect way a statement of unendurable stress; but they may not have any insight into what has caused such breakdown in ego functioning. Everybody has his or her level of stress tolerance, depending on the degree to which his ego experience has enabled him to bend rather than break. Stress up to this level can have much positive value: many goals are reached under great but not intolerable stress.

The severely emotionally deprived children I shall be considering in this paper have a very low level of such tolerance. The skilled and deeply concerned grown ups who care for them can tolerate considerable stress before reaching breakdown.

The ability to communicate stress even in retrospect can help to raise the level of stress tolerance both for the consumers and the providers of primary experience. I use this term 'primary experience' to refer to experience belonging to the first year of life, without which integration as an individual is impossible. Primary experience may be given to the baby by the mother-figure, or may be offered at a later date by the therapist.

A group of people working with emotionally deprived children in a residential setting are extremely vulnerable. They are working in an involved and undefended way; only thus can they provide the primary experience needed. In this paper I shall only be considering grown ups and children *inside* the residential place. The problem of communication to outsiders is too big to consider here.

I do not consider that there can be a satisfactory emotional economy in a staff group in which there is no direct intercommunication of stress. Because realization and statement can make stress *thinkable*, i.e. containable (since through realization the underlying cause of the stress may become conscious), the insight gained may be available on later occasions.

A group of people working together in a residential place come to know the best and the worst in each other: they often meet (at meal times, for example) when one or more of the group may be in a state of great tension; the degree to which such a state can be communicated to others will depend on the emotional climate in the group.

Sometimes stress may be displaced, often from people to things: so that, for example, instead of bursting into tears over some awful experience with a child in a rage, the worker under stress may complain with tremendous force about the weather, or the food, or anything else.

Sometimes the whole group can sit eating in gloomy silence; in fact they are slowly recovering from stress. A newcomer, arriving for lunch on her second day's work at the Bush, commented, 'It was as though a dark cloud hung over the table – I didn't know what to do!' An alternative to this behaviour is for the group to make a flight to reality, chatting briskly at a surface level, while stress continues to churn around beneath. Sometimes, when the group is not too stress-loaded, one or more members can communicate their desperate state of what is often emotional impoverishment following too much tension. On these occasions other people in the group may be able to empathize with the sufferer. Reassurance is useless, of course, and only makes matters worse.

Here I am talking about the aftermath of stress. Often this is

3

the only bit of the iceberg which is visible: we can but guess as to the real cause. By the time the stress is communicated, censorship may be seen in action. The worker communicates as much as he can bear to tell others without too much damage to his morale, prestige, or narcissism.

Winnicott, writing about the management of regression, points out that the strain involved is simple. I feel that we can make a useful distinction between *simple* and *complex* stress. Simple stress could be thought of as stress uncomplicated by guilt or other factors. For example, the stress experienced in sitting up all night with a child in a regression can be felt and communicated without guilt. If the child asks 'Are you tired?' the worker can reply 'Yes, I'm tired but I'm all right.' The circumstances of a regression are similar emotionally to those of early babyhood. The child is totally dependent on the therapist: the therapist is deeply involved with the child; and feeling something which is comparable to primary maternal preoccupation. Perhaps one of the most important characteristic features of such preoccupation is the lack of guilt. The ordinary devoted mother does not feel guilty in devoting herself to completely give to the needs of her baby; other people must take over her usual responsibilities for the time being: her stress is what I am describing as 'simple'. The worker involved in a regression has much the same experience, relying on colleagues to take over functions to enable him to sustain the role necessary for the child's regression.

If, however, a worker has been used (for example) as a reliable bad object through a long and exhausting evening by a very disturbed and testing child, then the worker may reach a stress level of angry resentment. He knows that if he is 'bad', another worker is probably 'good'. He is aware that this is a typical phenomenon at a certain stage of recovery; that he is doing valuable work by being reliably 'bad': yet because of the irritation and resentment at being used in this sort of way (for too long, perhaps) his state of stress is complicated by guilt. He is not sufficiently involved with the child for primary preoccupation to deal with the guilt (by projecting super-ego elements), so that he is not facing the simple stress I have described in connection with regression, but complex stress because of guilt experienced in respect of anger and resentment felt towards the child. These are feelings which the worker would wish to disown; and which he may deny, repress or displace so that the resentment may turn up in some other area of experience. Simple stress is therefore fairly easy to communicate; but complex stress is another matter, because of the element of guilt or other factors which may not be conscious.

Many people coming into this field suppose that a good worker does not become cross, or frustrated, or tired. They consider that a professional view is an objective one; that a professional worker remains calm and detached; that the measure of skill and experience can be judged by the degree of such detachment. Unless they happen to have had a personal analysis they may suppose that analysis ensures this emotional equilibrium; that an analysed person does not experience stress. This confused attitude often leads the inexperienced worker to adopt a facade – a false-self defence. Such a worker often does his best to disguise stress, to present a calm, untroubled front in all circumstances; to communicate happenings, however devastating, in a cool and apparently objective manner; and above all, to avoid describing his own feelings in regard to such experiences. When in a discussion group, a student using this defence is likely to be shocked and disconcerted by other more mature workers' communication of anger, fear, or distress. He will speak of such reporting in a critical way, often suggesting that to talk in this way is evidence of emotional disturbance.

We are evolving[1] a type of reporting at the Mulberry Bush which attempts to avoid pseudo-objectivity, and to help us to accept the fact that happenings do not take place in isolation; that we are also involved, and that we can never observe without observing a situation observed (if we watch a mother bathing her baby, we are watching this happening *when observed*; even our presence alters the happening in many ways). The type of reporting to which I have referred implies an acceptance of the contribution which we may make to a situation, even though we may not say or do anything.

Parents are often unable to understand how much they contribute to their children's emotional state by stress which is not

---

[1]Since this paper was written, this technique has been established.

directly communicated to the child by words or actions. For example, a baby can catch his mother's depression: the symptoms which he may then develop may never be traced to their source. Very often, if we are able to tolerate insight, if we can dare to know that we are functioning under stress, we can then communicate our feelings to children directly, instead of (for example) projecting such feelings on to them; when we are angry with taking responsibility for our own feelings.

I have often mentioned an episode which made a deep impression on me during the first years of 'the Bush'. I was sitting on the steps leading down into a dormitory full of restless, hot children at about ten o'clock on a summer's night. I was waiting for the children to go to sleep, and becoming more and more frustrated, irritable and desperate as the time dragged on towards darkness. I tried to read – I had brought one of Freud's papers to occupy myself – but the children kept on murmuring and chattering to me and each other. They explained that they kept on talking because if they were to stop, I would go downstairs.

I grew more irritated, trying without success to read my book, and finally spoke very sternly to one of the talkers. 'Be quiet!' I said. 'It's late – very late, and there is to be no more of this.' I tried to sound calm and collected; the children knew better. Presently after a brief silence, one of them asked 'What *is* the matter with you?' I replied that I was hot and tired and cross. Whereupon the questioner said, 'Well, why don't you go downstairs and read your book, and let us go to sleep.' I accepted the offer and the children went to sleep at once: they had been acting out my hidden anger and frustration for me. Disturbed children are highly intuitive: they react in any adverse way to pseudo-objective responses from adults, often picking up the underlying stress.

Inexperienced workers such as I have described run into grave difficulties of this kind, often because they think that to be permissive is always to be therapeutic. The outcome of pseudo-objectivity and false professional calm and detachment tends to be major or minor breakdown, sometimes into panic states or psychosomatic symptoms. It can be important to realize that anger, hate or anxiety, when acknowledged and communicated, are far less likely to be acted out either by ourselves or through the children; and that a child can be deeply reassured by the discovery that, on occasions, we may even hate him, but that this does not mean that we *withdraw concern* from him – we continue to try to meet his needs.

Children can sometimes communicate stress in a vivid way. Peter, a six-year-old at the Bush some years ago, described to me how he felt when furious with somebody whom he was afraid to attack. He said, 'It feels dreadful – like as if I'm a hedgehog with the prickles sticking *in* instead of out.'

Tom, a thirteen-year-old delinquent, communicated an experience of extreme stress, in retrospect twenty-four hours later. He explained: 'I felt queer inside, especially in my stomach. It made me think of what you said about excitement and pinching – the feeling was excitement. I've often had it, but didn't think of it like that. I thought I'd buy some sweets: I went to the tuck shop, but it was shut. The feeling got worse: I sat on the edge of my bed, I didn't know where to put myself. I had a shower, but it didn't do any good. Then I thought of roller skates, but there wasn't anyone to lend me a pair. I went on getting worse, then someone came back and let me use his skates. I went very fast, specially round corners. I got better: the feeling went'.

Stress frequently produces physical symptoms; the nature of which can help us to understand the deeper cause. I asked Tom whether he thought there could be a connection between the awful feeling and something that could have happened in babyhood. I described a baby getting desperately excited waiting for his mother to feed him, and his mother not coming at the right time, and the baby getting more and more excited; by the time she did come Tom interrupted at this point, exclaiming, 'He wouldn't want the *feed*!' I said I thought that the baby would be hungry, but that the excitement and splendid greed would have got split off from the food, where it belonged; and that if this often happened, such a baby would lose excitement connected with food, and feel it elsewhere not connected with anything, as free-floating stress. I suggested that his delinquency was a way of dealing with this isolated excitement, and that perhaps it might be possible to link excitement to food in some way. He told me that he was never interested in his food. We then worked out a plan together which would help him.

I have quoted this episode in some detail because Tom's undefended communication of stress made it possible to give him
much needed therapeutic help. If Tom has not been able to allow
me to know about what was going on inside him, I could only
have guessed at the nature of the problem. The fact that he could
give me an accurate description of stress in action within him
showed me the nature of this stress and enabled us both to understand the task ahead; the need to link the excitement with food,
where it originally belonged, instead of delinquent activity.

Jenny made a deeply felt protest against complex stress. She
needed at one time to cry, and for her crying to be accepted as a
direct communication of anguish. However, some workers found
her grief intolerable, giving her reassurance and trying to cheer
her up, instead of accepting this communication of sorrow and
pain. Jenny tried to adapt to these demands, but was too distressed to succeed. She said to me: 'I do wish people wouldn't
cheer me down.' This was a vivid description of an attempt to com-
plicate stress by mechanisms of flight or denial.

There are other contexts in which grown-ups find acknowledge-
ment of stress intolerable. For example, the kind of collusion
which goes on when a grown-up has to inflict pain on a child,
saying 'There's a brave boy!' instead of 'I'm sorry I had to hurt
you so badly': the boy has to be stoical because of the grown-up's
needs.

Johnny cut his hand and had to have stitches in the Casualty
Department of a large hospital. There was a lot of pain involved
which he bore with a terrible stoicism. This was troubling to
Vanno, a member of the Bush team, who was with him. The
doctor and the nurse congratulated Johnny on his courage—he
was now like a piece of granite—whereupon Vanno said quietly,
'Johnny, you do know don't you, that it's all right for you to
cry?' Johnny broke out into helpless sobbing, buried his head
in Vanno and collapsed. It is difficult for many people to understand that such breakdown can be necessary and therapeutic;
that without this communication of stress there will be trouble
later.

Much more common is the communication of stress in a more
disguised form, often by means of symbolization. Jeffrey, who
was epileptic as well as being severely emotionally deprived, came

8

to me in a very anxious state just after his arrival in the school. After several tentative questions he asked me whether I knew the rhyme of Humpty Dumpty. I replied that if Humpty Dumpty fell off the wall in the Bush we would try to pick up and hold all the bits. His relief confirmed my impression that he was speaking about his fits, which for him represented disintegration. Here is a symbolic communication of stress; which is, I think, usually best met by symbolic response.

In all these cases children have tried, fairly successfully, to communicate complex stress.

1. Peter, the hedgehog child felt prickles turned against himself, because he had to cope with aggression which he dared not express.
2. Tom's excitement had not been recognized by him as excitement, because this feeling was split off as a defence against intolerable waiting.
3. Jenny was able to continue her direct communication of simple stress because she was unable to make use of mechanisms of flight and denial.
4. In Johnny's case, grown-ups *needed* the child in pain to be stoical; as soon as he was given permission to feel hurt, he reacted in an emotionally appropriate way.
5. Jeffrey could communicate his stress in symbolic terms sufficiently clearly to be understood.

Children often express stress through non-verbal communication. They may scream, cry, cling, or become destructive: they may run away, climb a tree, or throw themselves on the ground. The response most likely to succeed is 'holding'; a technique used indiscriminately at Warrendale[1], but which can nevertheless prove valuable if used with discretion and in an appropriate context.

All of us are acutely aware of the dangers of institutionalization. Many of the children who come into our schools have been institutionalized following severe emotional deprivation during the first year of life. I think we can usefully consider the effect of institutional treatment on communication. One of the characteristics of severely deprived children is the inability to commu-

---

[1] Film: 'Warrendale', Allan King, 1967

nicate stress, which must nevertheless break through in the form of grossly deviant behaviour. An institution with a rigid organization forbids stress to be communicated. There is, as it were, a conspiracy to keep strong feelings below the surface, behind the facade of an institutional regime. Stereotyped phrases replace spontaneous communications, for adults and children alike.

There are often very dangerous subcultures in such places, but these are deeply hidden; collusive anxiety keeps them in the dark recesses.

I would suppose that systems of discipline in a place have a connection with the stress level which can be tolerated by the staff: the lower the level of stress toleration, the harsher the discipline. Organized and consistent (or rigid) methods of punishment, for example, tend to bypass conscious stress in the person who inflicts the punishment. Where there is 'punishment made to fit the crime' stress can easily be denied in a place. If a grown-up hits a child in a moment of anger, there is no escape from acceptance of some responsibility for both the action and the stress which led up to the action. This stress can be communicated to the child. Both grown-ups and children can gain from such experience, provided both are able to communicate their feelings to each other: because of the necessary insight involved, it is unlikely that such an episode will often be repeated. A person imposing disciplinary measures, however, often acts under considerable and complex stress of which he may not be aware. Both punisher and punished can be involved in a kind of unconscious excitement, which can result in a pairing set-up, and this may perpetuate a pathological punishing/punished pattern.

Professor Anthony in 'Group therapeutic techniques for residential units'[1] writes: 'The child very soon comes to know who wants to beat it and does not, who wants to treat it and cannot, and who imagines that he is treating it by beating it. The beaten child is learning slowly inside himself to become a beater.'

Psychotic children often turn out to be those who, because of having to endure intolerable and unthinkable stress, have withdrawn to a position in which they are able to believe that they

[1]Reprinted in Papers on Residential Work, Vol. 2 *Disturbed Children*, ed. R. Tod, 1968 p. 106

will never have to feel again. They may actually not feel stress, unless someone or something has broken through their massive defences.

Severely deprived babies often do not display overt indications of stress. They do not cry or rage, but remain passive and silent. Hospitalized children can be reduced fairly quickly to the same state.[1]

People working in this kind of setting tend to be so defended against awareness of their own and others' stress that they do not really come into close contact. with the children, nor with each other in relation to the children. We could say that a great deal of deprivation goes unrecognized because children have either lost or been forbidden the relief of communicating stress in a direct way; and this is often because the adult cannot stand the guilt involved in knowing the harm that has been and continues to be done.

One of the important areas in which symbolic communication of stress can take place is that of play: in fact children often deal with stress through play. When institutionalized children are concerned, there is no symbolic play; they cannot symbolize what they have not experienced (this applies to all really deprived children).

I hope that what I have said concerning the need for everyone to be able to communicate stress does not suggest that I am recommending masochistic orgies. Nothing could be further from my thoughts. I have already said that the level of stress tolerance varies from person to person. Many people—grown-ups and children—can contain considerable stress within themselves without difficulty. One has no right, I think, to invade the privacy of such people, who will be conscious of stress but able to deal with the problem themselves. What I *am* saying is that, if stress is above this safe level, there needs to be direct communication and sympathetic response. If such an exchange is acceptable in a group of people working with disturbed children, there are likely to be fewer headaches for grown-ups and fewer broken windows for children!

[1] James Robertson, *A two-year old boy goes to hospital,* Tavistock Child Development Research Unit, 1953.

Now and then someone turns up in a residential place who seems to thrive on stress. Usually one finds that this sort of person organizes stressful situations because he is, in a way, addicted to stress. I do not feel that such a person should be encouraged to communicate stress, but rather to work in some other field where the fulfilling of this compulsive need will not be so likely to damage others.

Ideally, we all would be able consciously to contain stress within ourselves up to a high level, understanding the causes – whether simple or complex – and not needing to defend ourselves against insight. Actually, however, because we are real people we cannot do this beyond a certain point; at which something must happen. It is not easy to recognize this danger point, so that often we defend ourselves against stress before we become conscious of feelings which may be surging up from very deep within us.

Rage or terror are likely to surface in a fairly recognizable form; but envy (about which Klein has taught us so much) can produce agonizing stress and yet remain unconscious. Even if we are conscious of envy this is a difficult form of stress to communicate, because nobody wants to acknowledge the feelings of inadequacy which envy implies.

Some time ago a skilled and experienced therapist worked for a year with us at the Bush: I shall refer to her as Emily. Emily was deeply involved with a difficult boy of ten called Paul. These two were going through a phase of Paul's treatment during which he was regressed to babyhood in relation to Emily. This regression was localized: Emily made special symbolic adaptations to his needs (such as Sechehaye describes), and in all sorts of ways was giving him primary experience which had been missing during the first year of his life. Emily was under a simple but continuous kind of stress which she could tolerate; she had the support and concern of the other members of the team who knew how important this regressed phase must be to child and therapist and who gave support to their therapeutic involvement.

Paul's mother had a new baby which she wanted to show to Paul, so Emily took him to see his home many miles away on a cold winter's day with an icy wind blowing down the streets of the slum in which he lived. Paul's mother was always maternally preoccupied with her babies during the first months of their lives;

as they began to separate out from her into people in their own right she rejected her children, they were no longer part of her. This is what had happened to Paul when he was a small baby, as soon as he was weaned.

Paul's mother welcomed Paul and Emily, but in a preoccupied way. She brought in the baby to show her son, and then fed it at her breast. From that moment onwards she seemed to cease to be aware of their presence, so absorbed was she with her baby. Eventually Emily said that they must go: Paul's mother, suddenly noticing her, exclaimed 'But it is very cold, you are not warmly enough dressed – I will lend you my coat!' In a daze, Emily accepted the coat, and she and Paul set out on the journey back to the Bush. She did not tell us what had happened until later: Paul seemed quite happy, Emily very tired, but next day she was ill with a fever, and most distressed. At first she could not bear to think or talk about what had caused her so much anguish; but as she gradually described the whole experience to me, we could see that she was in an acute stress, complicated by envy.

You will remember that Emily was maternally preoccupied with Paul in a conscious and therapeutic way. The experience she and the boy were going through together was illusionary (although really felt), but the mother/baby unity of Paul's mother and her new baby was real objectively and subjectively. Emily, therefore, who was essentially a maternal person, was suddenly attacked by desperate envy of motherhood. The therapist and patient in the course of provision of a regression were faced by the mother and baby in the midst of original primary experience.

Emily was not conscious at the time of feeling envy: she could remember being intensely cold (physically), neither in touch with Paul nor with the mother and baby, she felt isolated and excluded. When Paul's mother pitied her (I think that the mother's action was not motivated by *compassion*), offering Emily her coat, it was as though she was regarding Emily as a poor creature to whom she could give kindness; in this way she denied the value of the help which Emily was giving to her son Paul. Paul's role in all this was a further complicating factor. He seemed to have been projectively identified with the baby at his mother's breast; a projection which, of course, broke the slender thread of his link with Emily, intensifying her feelings of isolation and inadequacy.

The stress caused by Emily's unconscious envy had not been realized or communicated in time to prevent a breakdown into psychosomatic illness. Following her gain of insight and her communication to me, she could tolerate her envy, and made a rapid recovery from her illness. It is easy to see how intolerable it must have been for Emily to feel envy of the very person whom she felt to be responsible for her patient's deprivation.

The leader of a treatment team, be he head, principal, director, or warden, has to be sensitively tuned-in to evidence of stress among his team and among the children in his care. He needs sufficient courage and integrity on occasions to communicate his own stress to his team. John Armstrong, the Headmaster of the Mulberry Bush School, talked to an audience of people who work in special schools; he described some incident, finishing: 'And I looked at this child with hate, and he returned my look of hate. We both knew that we hated each other.' The troubled chairman asked John whether he was sure that he had really felt hate. John assured her that his was so. His audience was grateful to him, and rightly so; they accepted an important communication.

Liz Greenway, at that time a member of the team, was talking to Ronnie (aged eight). Ronnie said to her, in sugary tones, 'You're so kind to me, Liz.' Liz replied, 'But I lose my temper with you, Ronnie, and you lose yours with me.' He could accept this correction of the sentimentality that is really denied hate: because Liz could stand reality, however awful, he could also.

It is important that anyone who is feeling persecuted, badly treated, overlooked, or devalued, should be able to talk about these feelings to someone who can respond without collusion. Often there may be an objectively real grievance somewhere; but in any case, however irrational such feelings may be they are terribly *real* to the persecuted one–be it grown-up or child. Just to be able to surface such feelings can sometimes make insight possible, so that the sufferer can sort out reality from projection (projection makes such stress complex). If a child says to me, 'No one likes me, everyone is on to me', I would be likely to say, 'How awful you must be feeling', because it is the *feeling* he is talking about and this is real. I think one can neither usefully argue nor reassure on these occasions. A grown-up, however, who constantly feels persecuted is at risk in working with disturbed children; the kind of person who can say with James Payn (1884):

> I had never had a piece of toast
> Particularly long and wide
> But fell upon the sanded floor,
> And always on the buttered side.

I have written in this paper for the most part about individuals communicating stress, directly or indirectly. I shall now turn finally to group intercommunication under stress.

Miller, writing in 1960 about the use of small groups for staff training in the penal system, stated: 'Thus psychologically un-trained staff are constantly exposed to the psychological stress of being in interpersonal situations with highly disturbed human beings.' Individuals under this strain naturally bring their stress into group situations. I have for a long time been concerned with the problem of enabling workers to include their own feelings in reporting and group discussion. I started to wonder about 'the situation' in residential treatment as comparable to 'the session' in psychotherapy. I thought that 'the situation' needed to involve experience between the reporting adult and a child or children: an experience which was felt, recognized and realized, and com-municable to others.

This idea gradually evolved into what I have called 'context profiles', a kind of reporting which makes use of experience (rather than observations) between staff and child in the course of a week, at all times of the day and night.[1] Clare Winnicott, in 'Communicating with children',[2] writes: 'Shared experiences are perhaps the only non-threatening form of communication which exists.' I feel that *reporting* on shared experience can also be fairly non-threatening in an undefended group.

Here I am only going to consider a fragment of a group dis-cussion following the accumulation and recording of such a context profile, which had already been read by the team. I think this is an interesting discussion. Matters to be considered are: the stress involved; rivalry between the various people helping

---

[1] Papers on Residential Work, Vol. 3 *Therapy in Child Care*, chap. 10.
[2] Papers on Residential Work, Vol. 2 *Disturbed Children*, chap. 7.

this child; feelings of inadequacy and guilt in respect of the limited amount that we have been able to do with this very ill boy; frustration in regard to his capacity for group disruption – anger and disappointment; envy in regard to earlier workers (with whom present workers may be unfavourably compared). Because the team are individually and collectively acutely aware of such stress factors, their communication is not hampered or stereotyped.

David had been in the children's department of a mental hospital before he came to us, as one of the most deprived children I have met. He was at that time unintegrated in most areas. There was a very frail ego (built on such good experience as had come his way in babyhood and early childhood). In a few areas, therefore, he could function; for the rest, he was chaotic, needing almost total emotional containment. I think our discussion will explain more about him.

John: What I could not help but notice in reading all this was the lack of involvement with David which there seems to be: some of the notes I put in were really to indicate what David is doing now and what he is not doing, compared with a year or so ago.

Myself: Wouldn't you say that possibly this is because David is a running concern–you know, that he has a kind of outfit? This certainly seemed to me to come out in my session with him today. I seem to find this also in the material. To me there is the David who is tough, the bully, who attacks, who goes for people; and there is also the David who plays the recorder really beautifully. He played it to me this afternoon–he asked in the session if he could play it to me– and it was most moving: the delicacy of his fingers, the way in which he holds the recorder.

The contrast between this and the way in which he normally uses his fingers is tremendous. I feel there are these two aspects of David which, in a way, shut him off from the other people a bit, unless one can contact the part of him which plays the recorder. That's why one is in difficulties about getting close to him.

John: In a way I don't know how it has struck other people, but it seems to me that in the last fortnight the outward David is not what we have had. There has not been nearly so much beating up and sly kicking. How much all this has got to do with the recorder I don't know.

Myself: Well really the recorder is just a symbol. . . . I am just using the recorder as one aspect of his personality.

Hans: There is an apparent transition to a next stage, quite consciously over a long time. I feel I've had a long period making a primary provision. The fact that he came to me was more because he was making an attempt now into entering a suitable course of work.

Myself: Or secondary experience?

Hans: Yes. And as far as *I* have observed I think it has happened.

Myself: May I interrupt just a minute? There is Liz, and before her there was Faith, and one or two people in between . . .

John: Tita and Gillah briefly in between . . .

Myself: Yes, that's right. So that in fact there has been a sort of chain of mother figures that really now must be fairly strong and . . .

Liz: Mothers?

Myself: Yes indeed, mothers.

Liz: You may remember it was where I spoke of David preparing to leave my group to go over to that of a man, and making tentative approaches, looking for a father figure. He tried to make some connection with Hans in a magical sort of way. I have noticed how magic or apparent magic and power mattered so much to him, as if to make up for inadequacies in my maternal provision.

Myself: This makes very interesting sense of his recorder, doesn't it? As one could suppose that the making of music is a kind of symbolization of the early experience with you.

Liz: He wanted me to get him a transistor. And he wanted me to teach him to play the recorder. I was unable to teach him because I knew nothing of playing the recorder, and Hans was able to help him. My failure here was important.

Myself: This gives one the maternal history, so that learning lessons and so on are based on a masculine identification: learning the recorder has go to do with fathers.

Liz: But you will remember where I said that David has told me his father was Greek; that I would not be able to spell his name, that I would not be able to write it in Greek and so on.

Myself: One wonders what Greek means to David, if it has a real significance.

Liz: And he was asking how many words one could make from his surname, and about when he was born.

Myself: Apropos of his being born. Today at the very end of the session I was reminding him of how he talked to me about his birth (I met him in the very early days at the Limes[1]—I was trying to work out just how long ago this was) and how he described to me that he had been dropped in fact from an aeroplane on to bare ground, and had lain there till his mother found him.

John: I think his father was an airman.

Myself: That fits, doesn't it? . . . there he was on the hard bare ground and suddenly his mother came along . . . he says he remembers being found. Extraordinary, isn't it? It is relevant here to what happened in the session. He said that he would like to play squiggles—I couldn't remember if he was a squiggle child—however, he said that we had played squiggles.[2] There were three squiggles in this particular game, but I shall only describe two. David turned my squiggle into a large tangled sort of bow: then suddenly, down in the corner of the paper, he drew a rather beautiful form, a little like a tudor rose or a medallion—very small and precise. David said: 'That's a big bow, but this is what I really wanted to make.' I said cautiously that it looked to be more like a flower, but he didn't take it up. I was thinking really that here was this great big thing which he called a bow, but which looked to me very like a knot, and down here was this very small, neat, collected little thing which I thought was terribly important. I thought again here of the two aspects of David, and here they were: but I didn't say so.

David described the third squiggle: 'There are two planes signalling, one close and one far away.' I said I wondered what they were signalling to each other, and David said he didn't

---

[1] The Limes is a staff house.

[2] 'Squiggles' is a technique which I use with children, in which I make a small squiggle on a piece of paper, the child turns the squiggle into anything he likes. and we discuss the result.

know. I said I wondered why it was important, and David said: 'Well, they are both signalling to each other—I don't know what about.' I asked: 'Do they understand each other? This is the important thing—that they should understand one another—then it doesn't matter that other people do not know what it is about.' A discussion followed in which I made suggestions based on this and on the second squiggle, that these were (or could be) two parts of him. So he said: 'What nonsense! There is only one of me, you can see I am one.' I answered that I did see, but I didn't know if I could feel like David about him. So then we talked about this and he said: 'What do you mean?' I talked about the bully, boss part of him and all that, and he said was I sure I wasn't thinking about Tom. So I said I really was quite sure that I was thinking about David. He was extremely resistant, at first taking the line that anybody could see that there was only one of him: I agreed that this was all that could be seen, but I did feel there were two different parts of David as a person. He disagreed, and then I asked whether the part of him that is bossy knew about the part of him for whom Faith used to make custard. He said at once, 'No', and I suggested that this could be confirmatory evidence that the two parts of him were out of touch with each other. There is the part of him that plays the recorder and there is also the part of him that Faith used to make custard for . . . We talked about the recorder and the custard; this being a way of talking about parts of him. I said: 'Does this still sound nonsense to you, or does it make any kind of sense?' And he said, no, it didn't sound like nonsense to him, he was thinking about it. I said that if this was so, perhaps one could imagine that the tough bullying part was really protecting the little real part—I said that the recorder part seemed to be the real part.

I saw a great change in the description of what he had done with the recorder, and it did seem to me to confirm very much the fact that he is trying to give his real self a voice.

John: There is the fact that he would time after time go away to the sitting room and play.

Myself: There are lots of descriptions all through the context profile: the recorder is the clue to this boy.

Brian: This recorder: at times when he is threatened, say by Tom, he uses it in a way as a snake charmer would charm a snake. But of course, it does not have this effect. It is fascinating, he is not looking at the recorder, he is looking at the boy.

Hans: Of course I knew that David had started the recorder with Royston. When he came into my group he wanted me to continue because he knew I could, but I refused because I felt in this case it was too important–though occasionally he would ask me something to do with his music. I think it is a good sign that he is able to keep a rapport with a special person.

Myself: Yes, it is also conscious, and you will have to consider this in thinking about his establishing a father; he is building up his father from a selection of people: as he has also in a way built up a mother from a selection of people. The way things have worked out, this is how he is able to do it. The amazing thing is the amount he has achieved because of the group of people trying to work in the same way and doing the same things for him. He has shown me–and this is very interesting– he has shown me the other recorder: he got it out of the drawer. I asked: 'Is that all right, do you think?' and he said, 'Oh yes, just to show you and then put it back, that's all right–you tell Roy.' I said that I would. So he took it out of the drawer and showed it to me. He said: 'It's beautiful, quite beautiful. But it has got to get moist quite gradually. It would be awful if it just became what is called a "hoarse" recorder. This wouldn't make a nice sound–it would be loud and horrible.' I thought to myself–I didn't say this–just like David's voice when he is tough and horrible.

I felt there were two voices, and the recorder really was the voice of the real David . . . the David struggling to grow.

Liz: Do you remember how sensitive he was to voice, and he got so annoyed when I tried to read a story to the group with expression. He would say 'Read it in your own voice.'

Even in this fragment of a context, there is evidence that the speakers have dealt, and are dealing, with considerable stress.

1. At the beginning John drew attention to the lack of involvement with David, who has been with us for several years. John and all of us had felt guilt and anxiety about this fact, but neither John nor any of us denied the realization in order to

attempt to preserve an emotional equilibrium.

2. Hans told us that he had to provide David with primary experience when he first joined Hans's group. He pointed out that this provision was not completed in Liz's group, but that now David is able to go on to secondary experience. Hans had long since dealt with conscious resentment in regard to providing for someone who was so out of step with the rest of his relatively integrated group.

3. Liz was able to speak of inadequacies in her maternal provision, instead of blaming someone else or denying her failure. She went on to show that her failure in connection with David's learning the recorder could in fact be used by David. She could tell us that Hans was able to offer David something that she could not. A little later she speaks of David pointing out her deficiencies. All this could have been denied or projected, and be simmering under the surface.

4. I felt guilty and unhappy about David, because I had worked with him quite a lot when he first came to us. For various reasons I had lost touch with him. Now I felt a need to link past and present both in my own work and that of the others. In talking with David and the team I felt better as I realized just how much other people had achieved.

5. Hans, a very musical person, left the teaching of David's recorder to Royston, outside the group. This cannot have been emotionally easy to do; but he was concerned as we all were with the primary task of helping David. (We tend to work in terms of main and supplementary roles.)

6. Liz, at the end, mentioned that David liked her to read 'in her own voice'. This is the sort of wounding thing that disturbed children say, which can easily be felt as an attack on the worker. Liz did not make this mistake; she could tolerate the pain of being criticized or despised by a child.

7. We were all able, at different points during the whole discussion, to refer to earlier members of the treatment team who had helped David. Such reference is always emotionally loaded, because we are all having to accept the idealization by children of workers who have left; while we ourselves are angry with these people for going away. The fact that we know we are angry and have talked about our feelings frees us to value what

they have done and to miss them.

I have attempted in this paper to consider some of the many problems arising in the communication of stress.

I think we must accept that in the course of the residential treatment of severely disturbed children we are bound to encounter more and higher degrees of stress than would otherwise be likely to come our way. There will be times when the level of this stress will be higher than can be tolerated and contained. I consider that there will be less harm caused to ourselves and others if such intolerable stress can be communicated, rather than hidden or disguised. This communication cannot take place except among people who can acknowledge stress in themselves and are consequently able to be undefended and in empathy with others.

2

Emotionally deprived
parents, 1969

The therapeutic management of emotionally deprived parents
whose children are in residential treatment

I have always of necessity and of choice worked with the parents of disturbed
children. This particular paper was written for a course run by Chris
Holtom at Bristol University for child care officers, probation officers,
and others. My audience gave many interesting examples of experiences
with deprived parents.

I am finding difficulty in starting to write this paper, because I
cannot decide where to establish a beginning. I am going to make
basic assumptions concerning *your* starting point: I am going
to assume that most of what I might say has already been experienced, realized and conceptualized by all of us, so that I could
be wasting our time in covering a well tilled field.

There is a considerable collection of literature on the whole
subject of separation of children from their families, with which
I am sure you are already familiar; so that I propose to narrow
down the subject to certain special considerations which could
perhaps be interesting to discuss together.

We are all one way or another concerned with the effects of
severe emotional deprivation in parents and children, and with the
phenomena of 'acting out' which stem from a breakdown in
communication. At a time of crisis – such as can lead to the placement of a child away from his family – emotional deprivation (if
present to any extent in the child or the parents) can lead to violent
acting out, through breakdown in communication both with the
self and others.

The people in a residential place, be it approved school, maladjusted children's school or children's home, may be suddenly
confronted with a massive bloc of deprivation; which can have
serious effects on grown ups and children alike. How best we

can deal with this confrontation is what I wish to consider here.

In the therapeutic school where I work, we are selecting cases entirely on a basis of severe emotional deprivation during the first year of life. This being so, we have had to evolve a plan for admission which will avoid a sudden and tremendous build up of stress for ourselves, the parents, and the child.

Because children are referred to us from child guidance clinics, we are in a position to make the whole process of separation from the family and admission to the school fairly gradual. We start with interviews at the clinic, followed by one or more visits to the school. Eventually the parents bring the child to the actual placement, to people and a place already fairly familiar. There have, however, been occasions when we have admitted an urgent case from one moment to the next. I am sure that such a course of action is traumatic, but must become necessary in many cases where a child is committed to an approved school, or has suddenly to be taken into care because of some family catastrophe. On the whole, our small customers at the Mulberry Bush have been living in a state of endemic crisis, without total breakdown having taken place. Home, therefore, however pathological, continues to exist, thus making a gradual process of placement possible. Because deprived children tend to be the children of deprived parents, we can assume an absence of transitional experience in their lives: the filling of gaps in their emotional experience must be our primary task, and 'bridging' techniques in placement procedure can make a foundation on which we can hope to build, in providing primary experience.

The sudden removal of a child from his family, however pathological, is likely to be traumatic, and to reproduce previous traumatic breaks in the continuity of the child's existence which have led to his present state. Nothing can be more likely and more traumatic than such faithful reproduction for child and parents of earlier disasters, in the residential setting. There are circumstances in which there is no alternative, where transitional techniques cannot be employed, and the break between child and family has to take place from one moment to the next: at least we can be aware that this is something terrible, even in cases where there may be cruelty and neglect.

It is important to realize that the parents of severely emotionally deprived children are likely to be themselves deprived, even though this may not be immediately apparent from histories or initial interviews. One is liable to expect envy and hostility from the parents of disturbed children, arising from their feelings of inadequacy in having to allow outsiders to care for their children. This kind of reaction is certainly to be expected from the parents of neurotic children: in cases of deprivation the problem is rather different. Parents in such cases feel envy also, but they are envious not of us, but *of their own children*, because their children are receiving the care which they know themselves to need. Once we become aware of this particular form of envy, we are already in a position to establish a link with the child *and* his parents (as compared with casework with individuals). It is possible to make limited provision for deprived parents, in terms of communication, food, time, and so on.

We are going to have a difficult task, in any case, in attempting to preserve the child's place in the family. If we start our programme by breaking the continuity of the family life by a *sudden act of separation*, we are certain to have much more difficulty than we need expect. If we can link both parents and child to us and the place, by localized provision before the child is actually placed, we may be able to replace an *act* of separation by a *process*; which, though sad and painful, need not be inevitably traumatic and can establish a bridge between family and place. Psychiatric social workers, health visitors, child care officers, teachers and probation officers can all play a part in this process, by acting as catalysts through whom the child and his family can come into communication with the people in the place (be it children's home, school for maladjusted children, or approved school). This assumes that the main catalyst agent is already in touch with the people in the residential place: this would seem to be essential in any case.

Deprived people, both grown-ups and children, have usually had to shift their trust from people to things: environment, therefore, can offer either security or threat. The unknown environment tends to be the threatening one, and I have known deprived parents and children to disorientate completely in going round our school for the first time. One must provide families with a base, a 'safe place' from which to explore the strange milieu. This base needs, I think, to be a sitting room of some kind, in which they can talk with members of staff, where they can have some food, and where they can be securely alone.

The illusionary 'safe place' will be a permanent need, because such people have no safe place within themselves. The 'safe place' can only exist at the price of other places being 'dangerous': if the safe place becomes less safe, the other places become more dangerous.

Initially, we ourselves combined with our residential environment will be felt as a dangerous place; so that by providing a family base we are preventing the child's family from starting their contact with us from a persecuted position. Of course we are hoping to establish relationships, but this is a long-term treatment aim. In working with deprived families, 'things' may come before 'people', just as acting-out is likely to precede communication.

What we *do* can in a symbolic way perhaps be more use than what we *say*, however relevant the latter may be. However warm a welcome we give to the family, what we feel and what we express may not reach them if the sun is not shining or if the room is cold. The hot cups of tea may convey this warmth, evoking what Sechchaye has described as symbolic realization.

When we are trying to help neurotic people, we can assume that they will transfer this and that on to us from their own early experiences; so we may become established in all sorts of roles which do not often have much to do with what we really are like as real people. We accept such roles, but do not act out *in* the roles; we keep these within the framework of our particular functions.

Working with deprived parents and children, we may be having very different responsibilities and commitments, since for them there can be no transference in areas where they have not had experience. This state of affairs leads to what Little has called 'delusional transference': for deprived people we *are* the parents— there is no 'as if' in such a feeling. It is all very well when such a delusional transference is positive, but when the negative form turns up, we can feel destroyed by the violence of annihilating rage which we may collect. Sometimes we may receive this terrible onslaught in the first place; more often we start with a positive delusional transference, in which we are the ideal parents who can take care at last of the parents *and* their children. They have been looking for such maternal care all their lives: so that if we reject these deprived fathers and mothers of deprived children, we confirm all that they suppose. On the other hand, we are in no position to take on full therapeutic responsibilities in relation to these families: it is their *children* who are our clients. Workers in a residential place recognize intuitively the needs of deprived parents, and realize how overwhelming would be their demands: so they tend to defend themselves against intolerable commitment, and in doing so tend to build a wall between themselves and the family of the child, who is now on the worker's side of the wall of defence.

What I am suggesting is the possibility of meeting the parents' needs in a highly localized way from the start. In fact we are much more likely to be able to give real therapeutic care to deprived parents than to neurotic ones, because *provision* rather than interpretation is the primary need. It is this fact that makes it possible for unanalysed therapists to learn this very special skill. The workers will need support and supervision; but they are quite likely to have sufficient personal resources at their disposal to provide appropriate therapeutic management in all areas for the deprived children, and in localized form for their parents.

People working with deprived parents tend to ask: 'How can we hope to help such damaged people?–how can the little we can do be of any use?' I think we can only reply as we would to the same question put to us concerning severely emotionally deprived children and adolescents: 'The ego is built of experiences. Therefore, in terms of strengthening a weak ego, we can be sure that no positive experience that we provide will be wasted.' This is a problem of economy, not of success or failure. We can only give what can be spared; but localized provision can be of value: parents and children can increase functioning areas through such provision.

I very rarely use the word 'adult', preferring to say 'grown-up'. 'Adult' seems to deny that *a child has grown up,* confirming the split which many parents and children feel divides them from each other. In recognizing the deprived child who has grown up into this unhappy and troubled parent, we can understand the unsatisfied and continued childhood needs of such a grown-up.

Talking about herself, a little patient of mine once said of her drawing 'This is a puddle in a pond'. The child hidden in the personality of the grown-up may be as secret as the puddle in the pond. The more well a mother is, the more linked she is with her own childhood, and therefore the more able to identify with her child's needs. If we can help the deprived grown-up to let us know about the hidden child with its desperate needs and to allow us to meet some of them (however small), we may be putting the mother in a position to feel for her child.

Of course, this is equally true of fathers, but because deep deprivation belongs to the first year of life we can assume that the mother is our first consideration, in the interests of her child. On occasions, however, the father has been the parent who has been able to feel maternal towards the baby, while the mother has been forced into a paternal role. Pathological though this is, we may have to be thankful that there is maternal feeling somewhere, and make use of what is available. In such a case we certainly cannot begin to alter the psychopathology of the parents. Here again, we must accept a very limited aim, but the little we *can* do may go a long way eventually.

It is a delicate task to help the deprived children in the personalities of the parents, whilst continuing to respect them as grown-ups, objectively speaking. However, we do respect as people within their own right the patients we are treating who are indeed *actually* children: similarly, we can soon perceive the functioning areas in even very deprived parents, where we can respect and support their maturity.

I remember, from long ago, a very disturbed father whose child was having a period of treatment in the Mulberry Bush School. We had come to know him quite well, and he was talking about his own need to come and be a child also in our care. He said, 'I wish I could do something here that I would do if I were small and living here.' I knew that he could draw very well, and suggested that he might paint a picture on a wall in the place. He was tremendously pleased, set to work sitting on the floor in the corner of a play room, and painted a fine ship—low down on the wall, at just about the height he would have been able to reach as a little boy. We could all (grown-ups and children alike) respect and admire his skill and the beauty of the ship; but at the same time we could sympathize with the child who was briefly among the other children in our care.

I have considered some ways by which parents may be linked to their residentially placed children, through their own localized experiences provided by the people in the residential place. I wish now to consider the more direct links between the deprived child placed residentially, and his parents.

Communication between the deprived child and his parents has probably broken down—if it has ever existed. There can, of course, be an institutionalized exchange of stereotyped phrases, but this is not real communication. The parents will react violently to the child's acting out, but are most unlikely to see this as attempted communication; indeed, they are liable to *re*act out themselves. We tend to think in terms of *maintaining* a link between child and home: but in the care of deprived family constellations, our task may well be to establish a link for the first time.

The telephone can be very useful: often this will be the first occasion on which child and parents have spoken to each other by telephone, and the very newness of the situation can break through the stereotyped conversation and lead to real communication. We explain to parents during initial interviews that we do not censor telephone calls or letters; so that (we point out) at first the child is likely to use this freedom to complain about us and other children. The deprived child will have learnt that his best chance of contacting his parents has been on a basis of persecution. This is the area where his parents can projectively identify with him, because they themselves will be paranoid in a very primitive way. If we can show children and parents that we can allow them to verbalize such complaints (which are often wholly irrational) without being hostile or punitive, we shall be making a start in the clearing of ground for communication in the family.

We have noted how often a child will hurt himself, or develop psychosomatic symptoms, or get himself attacked, just before the start of holidays. He is trying in his way to ensure a place for himself in the family to which he is returning and from which he has been excluded. He feels—usually correctly—that a persecuted niche is the only one on which he can count in his home, better this than nothing. Gradually we may be able to alter this dreadful pattern: sometimes this can be done by helping the child to bring back home something from the place—a bunch of flowers, a cake he has baked, or a stool he has made.

Both child and parents will be constantly threatened by a harsh projected super-ego: all authority will seem threatening and punitive to them. We are, for them, authority figures. They may adapt to our demands, but this will be placating and based on fear. When we try to meet their needs and care for them, we do not cease to be authority figures; but we can replace the harsh super-ego by a benign one. Of course we should like to be in ego-supporting roles, but for this to be possible there must be egos to support! Working with really deprived people (whether parents or children) we must learn to do without functioning egos in our clients: bits of ego there will be, but not enough.

We have been perhaps too willing, in the past, to decry the super-ego (the conscience arousing guilt and anxiety). The concept of the benign super-ego has not been so familiar. The acceptance of a parental authority role based on compassion and concern involves us in a different kind of involvement from the supportive role which is appropriate for work with integrated neurotic clients.

I recently had an initial interview in a child guidance clinic with the little son (aged eight) of psychotic parents: he was in care under Section I.[1] I shall refer to him here as Tommy. Both his parents could just about survive in society, but Tommy, a charming and intelligent boy, was breaking under the strain of widly inconsistent and unreliable management (he ran away from any placement, and from home). Discussing his problems with the psychiatrist, I gave it as my view that Tommy must be brought before a court as beyond parental control, so that he could be sent to us with legal controls. I suggested that if this plan could be accepted by Tommy and his parents, they might all feel more secure. Otherwise, I was sure, Tommy would be whisked away from us on impulse—either his own, or that of his parents. I wanted to establish authority between impulse and action. Accordingly, since the psychiatrist agreed with this line of thought, we discussed our ideas with the child and then with the mother; explaining our reasons, but in such a way that they were able to accept such authority, which was not felt by them as punitive (we have still

---

[1]Children Act 1948 (Section 1 makes provision for local authorities to receive children into care on a voluntary basis).

to learn the father's views).

I can remember several cases in which the children in treatment with us were making good progress, and we seemed to have a reasonably good contact with the mothers, albeit of a rather superficial kind. The fathers, however, stayed as shadowy figures in the background, both in regard to ourselves and to the clinics concerned: they appeared to accept what was being done to help their children, they did not participate but neither did they interfere. Suddenly, however, these fathers announced that their children must now come home. Nothing that any of us could do or say influenced this decision, and these children left us long before their treatment was completed.

However difficult the task of looking after these very disturbed people (be they grown-ups or children), their individual needs must somehow be met in very different ways. I think perhaps one's own attitude can make this easier. If one is working in a personal way rather than in an institutional way, the treatment approach can be flexible. If there is not too rigid an organization (in regard to visiting, for example) then there is not so much likelihood that the social structure will be disrupted by individual plans for parents' visits.

I remember a very ill mother, whom I met for the first time with her little daughter (aged seven) in a hospital department. The mother had tried to kill herself and her child, whom I shall call Polly. The hospital had offered to be responsible for both till other arrangements could be made—an offer which the court had accepted. There was a symbiotic tie of a most primitive kind between mother and child. I played squiggles with both of them together in their small bedroom, but I forget the exact details of this game. The mother was sure that she and Polly could not be separated, but she agreed, following a long discussion, to come and see the Mulberry Bush, brought by the psychiatric social worker. During this visit we played squiggles again; and between the two of them, mother and child produced from my squiggle a chicken coming out of an egg.

Polly came to us on condition that her mother could visit or telephone her at any time. Presently her mother started to tell me about her own life, and for the first time wanted to see me apart from Polly. I suggested that on these occasions we should meet alone in Oxford, to be joined later by Polly. In the Botanical Gardens we met on warm spring days, during which Polly's mother started to attack me—only with her voice—but in such a terrible way that I felt destroyed by her. I was often tempted to withdraw from the full blast of psychotic rage (the other face of her suicide attempt): but not to survive her 'destruction' of me would have been to take a terrible revenge upon her.

So our meetings continued, until one day she was telling me how vile we all were and how awful it was for her to have to leave Polly in our care, and that she had been forced by us to do so. I pointed out that there was no reason why she should have to leave her child with us—there were other schools—would she prefer us to make arrangements for Polly to go elsewhere? I held my breath at this point, but Polly's mother, having sat in silence for a moment, said slowly: 'She'd better stay at the Bush. There wouldn't be someone I could shout at, like I do at you, if she went somewhere else. Sensible people wouldn't stand for it!' On this basis Polly's treatment could continue, although eventually her mother removed her on an impulse.

What I am saying about deprived parents of children in treatment is that we cannot count on their evolvement. We may well have to accept them exactly as they are, have been and will be all their lives. We can nevertheless so gear our treatment programme as to make it possible to include them with their children in what we plan: should we fail to do so, they will certainly break into their children's treatment because of envy and feelings of rejection.

While a deprived child is in our care, we may ourselves be helping him to establish a place in his family *for the first time*. A neurotic child may be a square peg trying to fit into a round hole: a deprived child may have to evolve into a peg for whom we have to carve a hole—this can only be done on a basis of caring for the family as well as the child.

3
Integration and unintegration, 1969

This paper was written before chapter 5, 'Meeting children's emotional needs in residential work', so much that I have said here is contained in the later paper. However, I am including this short piece here because this is where I first stated my realization of the urgent need for classification in residential places.

I have felt for some time that the difficulty which most bedevils the residential treatment of disturbed and emotionally deprived children is the mixture of integrated and unintegrated in any one unit. The presence of such a mixture puts a terrifying strain on both staff and children, resulting in violent reactions.

The cornerstone of the ideas I am considering is this: I am sure that there is an enormous problem of *incompatibility*, with which integrated and unintegrated children are burdened if they are living together, and that this problem puts too heavy a load on staff. Those children who have not been able to establish a more or less functioning self are deeply threatened when confronted by functioning in others. They react to such a confrontation by a primitive defence which can be termed disruption (Erikson has applied this term to play). For example: if an unintegrated child comes into a group of integrated children who are playing an organized game, he will feel so threatened by the functioning children, he will at once attempt to disrupt (disintegrate) the group. The integrated children in the functioning group will become so anxious in the face of often repeated disruption that they will cease to make good use of their capacity to function and will, of course, feel bitterly resentful towards the disruptive ones, and towards the grown-ups who allow such disruption to take place.

The unintegrated children cannot stand functioning in others unless it is directed towards provision for themselves: the integrated children cannot stand constant disruption of their functioning as individuals or in groups. This is one kind of gross

33

incompatibility which can make life impossible for both kinds of children.

One can argue, of course (and rightly), that there are areas of incompatibility in all relationships. These areas can be denied or avoided, they can be battlefields, or they can be acknowledged and respected as unalterable (as they often are). Now and then in ordinary life settings, love and insight can bridge the gulf between the incompatible areas of two grown ups; but this is an achievement, because the causes for such incompatibility are so deeply rooted in the nature of the self, and the way in which the self has been built: this need not point to a lack of integration. The kind of incompatibility which I am describing is basic, in that one group is a threat to the survival of the other.

Another aspect of the incompatibility of integrated and unintegrated children is the incidence of panic amongst the unintegrated ones. Anyone, however integrated, is liable to panic for brief instants now and then, but unintegrated children panic constantly when emotionally they are *in a gap within themselves*. Panic can appear as rage, fright or despair: it can result in violent acting out or total immobilization. The therapeutic treatment of panic involves holding, containment, and very intensive care from a deeply involved therapist. Nothing is more difficult than to treat panic in the middle of a normally functioning group–at a meal time, or in a class, or play group, for example.

In order to make a classification of children in terms of integration, in a residential place, these two factors – disruption and panic–may be used to give some indication of the position. Clearly, in an approved school or a school for maladjusted children, there will be many more unintegrated children to be found in the group. I believe, however, that there is a high proportion–higher than we realize–of unintegrated children in children's homes and reception centres. A recognition of the effect which this presence must have on more integrated children and the people working in the place is a first essential step towards improvement.

Of course panic and disruption are not the only characteristics of unintegrated children, but these are overt symptoms which are quite easy to recognize and are reliable indications of unintegrated states. Once such a classification has been made, we are faced with problems of management. Would it be better for unintegrated children to be grouped together in special units that provide primary experience, or can the basic incompatibility of the integrated and unintegrated be bypassed within the one unit with special provision for the two groups? One argument (amongst many which would suggest the need for special units for unintegrated children) is that in, for example, a children's home, there may well be many more integrated than unintegrated children present. This is certainly the impression which I have received from listening to workers. It would be difficult to make special provision for, say, three out of sixteen children; the integrated children could suffer; the staffing ratio would not allow the amount of time and care needed for the therapeutic management of three children in a group of sixteen. There may be children's homes where there is a higher incidence of unintegrated children—perhaps six or seven in a group of sixteen: in such a case I would have thought that special management could be provided. Let us consider the possibilities in such a home. I am going to assume that all the children go out to school, and that the age range is from five to fifteen. The areas where special management could be needed would be meal times, bedtimes, the early mornings and play times. Bedtime always presents difficulties to unintegrated children, producing frequent panics, acting-out and disruptive activity, *unless* their needs are being met. Such children need to be cared for in the very special way I have described elsewhere:[1] for example, they need individually filled personal hotwater bottles (such a colour, so full, so hot—*this* bottle belonging to *this* child). They need special 'tucking in', and highly personal communication with the therapist worker concerned, once they are in bed. They may need a special kind of drink or sweet, their own cup, and so on.

Whilst it is possible to make such provision in a mixed group of integrated and unintegrated children, there are obvious disadvantages in doing so. For example, this could invite integrated children to regress when they have no need. If all the children sleeping in one room are unintegrated, they will each have their

---

[1] See 'The problem of making adaptation to the needs of the individual child in a group' in Papers in Residential Work, Vol. 2, *Disturbed Children*, 1968.

35

own provision and will be as unconcerned by the presence of other children as babies would be. The integrated children would then be free to read, talk or go to sleep in a peaceful atmosphere, instead of being disturbed by the panics and disruption which can lead to such bitter resentment and retaliation. The staff would be in a position to meet needs in an appropriate way, rather than struggling through intolerable and unresolved difficulties which arise from a mixture of grossly incompatible groups.

Meal times are another area of difficulty, and here perhaps two or more tables could help both groups (with three or four children at each table), thus avoiding a mixture of groups. Food is an essential field for primary provision: such a plan could make special arrangements feasible for the unintegrated, and which the integrated children would not in fact want for themselves.

Some of you may have read my suggestions for two types of play group,[1] one type assuming ego functioning, while the other would provide containment and primitive satisfactions.

Although I have not suggested acting out as a factor for classification, I wish to consider this typical phenomenon of unintegration from the viewpoint of provision. Acting out can be assumed to have resulted from a breakdown in communication. The re-establishment of a field of communication is therefore an important therapeutic task. Here again, in a mixed discussion group there will be disruption and panic for obvious reasons. Separate groups of integrated and unintegrated children can, however, function successfully and can lead to communication replacing acting out as unintegrated children learn to contain and verbalize their feelings. During the early stages of such communication, a flow of persecuted accusations are to be expected and accepted: that is to say, the reality of the persecuted feelings–not the validity of the accusations–must be accepted. It is easy to be trapped into proving how unreal these accusations seem to be; but in proving the point the therapeutic benefit of such communication can be lost.

I believe that in all units these small discussion groups should exist, taking place in the same room at the same time each day. The integrated ones will, of course, make use of such an opportu-

---

[1] 'Play as therapy in child care', in *Therapy in Child Care*, ch. 11

36

nity in quite a different way, but they also need a chance to talk in this special setting.

Ideally, in a mixed unit of integrated and unintegrated children there should be two 'quiet rooms'; one intended for functioning children, where they could read, paint or play quiet games without constant threats of disruption, and the other providing containment for non-functioning children, with large boxes, cushions, soft toys, blankets, etc. One room could be termed 'the quiet room club', with elected members, while the other could be called a 'box room', or some such name, which would not stress the real purpose for this room; its purpose could then emerge naturally as children started to use the facilities offered.

So far I have only discussed the management of a mixed group (in terms of integration) within one unit. The other possibility for consideration is the setting up of small residential units, catering only for the needs of unintegrated children. (Such a plan could easily exist in a 'cottage homes' arrangement.) If these special units could be set up, a flexible system would need to operate, by which children could move in and out according to their needs. These special units would require a high staff ratio (one grown-up to two children), and the staff would receive special training. Within the Cotswold Community (where I work) such a unit has already been in existence for long enough for us to see how well such provision can be used. The presence of this unit provides a valuable safety-valve, in that a disruptive, panicking actor-out can be referred to the special unit without imposing feelings of guilt and inadequacy on to the referring unit. It is now common for boys to refer themselves to the special unit, where primary experience is provided by a skilled team who have learnt the theory and practice of this kind of therapy in less than two years. The Mulberry Bush School caters only for unintegrated children, aged from five to twelve years. Here the presence of a recovering group of more or less integrated children presents a problem which has not yet been fully resolved. These recovering children have, however, themselves received the therapy of primary provision, so that they do understand to some extent the problems of the unintegrated children in treatment. But there is also a need here for more insulation, for a barrier against stimuli, to protect the newly established selves.

The ideas which I have put forward are based on limited experience and are only intended to provide a brief outline.

I have now been working at the Cotswold Community in a consultative role for nearly two years.[1] In common with other consultants, I was asked by Richard Balbernie, the Principal of the Cotswold Community, to try to find out for myself in what way I could be of use in the place. This flexible approach made it possible for me to feel my way, taking time and working in terms of the current context. What I have written up to this point are the conclusions I have reached with some certainty, so far: they are for the most part based on weekly discussions with the teams of the individual houses with which I have been connected. At first I did some work with the boys themselves, but I have found that I can be of more use to them indirectly—that is to say, working through the teams which help the boys. Anyhow, one session per week was hopelessly inadequate, and I found that the only way in which a single hour of psychotherapy could be of use was if it could be used afterwards for discussion with staff (of course, with the permission of the boy himself). Where unintegrated children were concerned, I pooled my resources with those of the staff, in order to work out a therapeutic programme of provision of primary experience for the particular boy—where I was, then and there. When working with an integrated boy, my main aim was to deepen the channels of communication between the boy and the staff caring for him.

The setting up of the small internal unit (known as the Cottage), explicitly planned for the provision of primary experience, took less than a year to establish as a functioning entity within the community. The speed with which the Cottage team learnt this highly skilled task astonished me, and made me think again about training in this field of work: I certainly had not realized how quickly a group of people *could* learn, in action. Perhaps learning as a group has advantages. The Cottage team has certainly come through deep and painful experiences in the course of realization about themselves in relation to the boys: I think that the outcome has made the difficulties and stress worth while. The team provides primary experience for the least integrated boys in the commu-

[1] This paper was written in 1969.

nity (about eight or nine); and also provides reliable support for each other, without which such work cannot be achieved.

In this group of boys there is no mixture of integrated and unintegrated, so that the problems are simple (those of the unintegrated) rather than complex (those of the integrated). Boys who achieve some degree of integration in the Cottage either leave the community or go back into the main stream of community life. Now and then a boy asks to see me, usually when he is nearing recovery, but this is unusual. The boys in the Cottage know what I do, and discuss this with the team. When the Cottage project was launched, I gave the boys a fruit bowl, which stands in their little sitting room, and which I fill each week with fruit: there are no rules about this bowl of fruit, and they like the idea— they do not exploit or spoil the arrangement, and they explain the idea to newcomers. In this way I can assure them of my concern, without interrupting the treatment process in the Cottage by impingement.

The other houses in the community face rather different problems: mixtures of integrated and unintegrated boys, and more staff changes, perhaps, than in the Cottage. In these houses I have similar discussions with the teams: always open discussions of any theme which comes to the surface, but always linking themes to specific happenings. As I slowly became aware of this concept of incompatibility, which I have been thinking about, it seemed urgent to help the teams to *classify* their respective groups in terms of integration. We used the two factors which I have already mentioned—panic and disruption—to make a rough classification within each house: we have tried to consider integrated and unintegrated children as two groups needing different kinds of therapeutic management. I am by no means sure that this is possible, but at least the task is being attempted. Eventually I would hope that units could be smaller, and that boys could be established in groups planned on a basis of integration and consequent compatibility.

All houses have, for some time past, made use of a morning meeting for all the staff and boys of each unit every day. Great difficulties have been experienced in establishing communication in these groups, because of disruption and panic phenomena, with considerable acting out and immobilization (resulting from a breakdown in communication). By breaking down this large house meeting into small groups (four in each) on a basis of degree of integration, communication has been established. We hope to bring the small groups together (each with the grown-up leader) to form an integrated whole, when we are confident that there is sufficient functioning for this to be possible.[1]

I believe that if we can think in these terms, some of our major problems in residential work may be at least partially solved.

[1] Actually, we have never taken this step, because the small groups function so well.

4

Communicating stress in
student supervision, 1969

This paper was read to a child care group, the members of which were all involved in student supervision. I feel that supervision of students in residential places is still sadly inadequate: a great deal remains to be thought out and properly structured in this area.

In chapter 1, 'Problems arising in the Communication of Stress', I discussed the communication of stress between deeply disturbed children and the adults who try to help them, in a residential treatment setting. I have been thinking a great deal about this subject, and want particularly to consider the problems attending the communication of stress by students and supervisors in relation to the supervision situation.

I recently read an interesting article by Janet Mattinson about the supervision of a student in a residential place by an outsider who knew both the student and the people who were running the place[1]. Reading this paper, I thought how fortunate are people who do their own supervision of students in a residential setting. Outside supervision is likely to cause splitting (between the people in the place and the supervisor) and an odd sort of collusion between the supervisor and the student, in regard to the people in the place.

Many students use their theoretical knowledge as a defence against having real experience. If they are being supervised from outside this becomes especially easy, because they can defend themselves against feelings of anxiety and inadequacy in the situation within the place, by intellectualizing what they are going through: so that they can in some way feel a conscious sense of superiority to the people in the place. It is difficult for an outside

---

[1] Janet Mattinson, 'Supervising a residential student'. *Case Conference*, April 1968, Vol. 14, No. 12.

supervisor to recognize this defence for what it is, a cover for anxiety. Where there is a supervisor inside the place (presumably one of the people who are in charge) such mechanisms become more obvious. For example, when a student in the therapeutic school where I work as a consultant says to the Head, 'Of course I am more likely to take an objective view of what is going on in the place than all of you who are so over-involved with the children', the Head is in a position to say, 'It must be awful for you, coming into a community like this, and feeling an outsider.'

Perhaps the real problem about the communication of stress is that people can very rarely report on what is happening inside them, except in retrospect. For example, a student who has, let us say, been in a panic state in regard to the management of a child's temper tantrum, may report on the tantrum as though he or she witnessed this quite calmly as an objective observer. Part of the trouble lies in the fact that the student, in common with many workers in the field of child care (and indeed, of all work with people) feels that to be professional is to be objective; and that the more detached, clearheaded and calm they appear to be, the more they will be accepted as a professional person. They are therefore liable to avoid talking much about how they really *feel* to their supervisors, in areas where they think that this may lead to critical judgements on their capacity as professional people.

It can on occasions be of value for the supervisor to be able to talk about his own experience of stress, in a way which helps the student to understand that realization and communication of stress make it manageable, and bring it within the total picture of what anyone experiences when working with other people. This may at first have the effect of shaking the confidence of the student in the supervisor; but gradually the fact that the supervisor is not alarmed or made to feel anxious or inadequate through the communication of stress may make it safer for the student also to talk about experience of stress. If the supervising person does not talk about his own difficulties in terms of experiencing stress, then the student is likely to be confirmed in his delusion that all professional people are invariably calm and detached in every situation.

It is interesting from this point to consider the *phenomenon* of stress. The extreme of this is panic, which has been described as 'unthinkable anxiety': it is the unthinkable quality which makes it impossible to communicate states of panic, except in very special circumstances. This is because unthinkable anxiety belongs originally to a pre-verbal era, when the baby who experienced something awful could not think about it but only feel, because he had no words with which to think.

There are, however, many degrees of stress which *can* be communicated; but it would seem vital that this should be as near the context as possible: communication will become more and more modified and rationalized in the passage of time. This makes me think that it is very important that students should be able to communicate to supervisors at all sorts of odd moments, rather than have an hour every week or a short time every evening, or any other such formal arrangement. The formal arrangement has its place, and an hour's discussion alone with the supervisor each week will be necessary and invaluable; the communication of stress is not so likely to turn up during such an hour as it is if the student knows that, in a moment when he is finding himself beyond his threshold of containable stress, he can come straight to the supervisor and talk about this, even if it is for only a very few minutes. The sheer *fact* of communication makes the stress tolerable, lowers the level of stress to where it can be contained; in other words, brings the stress within the particular threshold of the individual. The level of stress tolerance varies so enormously from person to person that this must be a highly individual matter. Flexibility in regard to communication can lead to a rising of this threshold in the individual, so that he will gradually find himself able to tolerate a higher degree of stress.

In recommending informal opportunities for the communication of stress I may be cutting across current ideas about the best way for supervisors to work, but I am deeply convinced about the importance of what I am saying, and you must consider my views for what they are worth, and discard them if you do not feel that they apply to your own work.

All of us inevitably do the sort of 'tidying up' I have described, in regard to our experiences; none of us can communicate really directly and honestly how we have felt and behaved in a particular context, if we have not satisfied our own standards in the situation. The longer we wait to discuss such adverse experiences which can be undermining to our morale the more likely are we to modify, distort, or alter what has happened to us. This is why I feel so strongly that immediate communication of stress is the only way in which such modification may be avoided, at least to a certain extent. This is especially true as the student gains confidence in the supervisor, because he is receiving sympathy and concern, rather than criticism and accusation, which is what he is expecting at first.

People have different aims when supervising students; obviously this must to some extent be so, because of the variation in the maturity and experience which the student brings to the placement. Some supervisors wish to impart as much knowledge, skills and techniques as may be practical in the particular setting. Other supervisors try to help the student to tolerate and gain some insight into the experiences which he communicates. Personally, I feel that knowledge, skills and techniques can only be used in a valuable way if they are based on experience, and realization of experience. Such experience is usually disturbing, and can raise the level of stress, and the student may avoid realization by one or the other of the defences which are at anyone's disposal; and, unless communication takes place, there may be an area of experience which the student may tend to avoid because it provokes anxiety.

Lisa, a student I was supervising, was experienced and clever. She brought me a happening for discussion.

Lucinda, a small patient of mine (of whom I have spoken before)[1], was building a little house for herself out of branches and leaves. Lisa found her trying to complete the house, and in some difficulty, particularly with the windows. Lisa offered to help, and in no time was established in the little house, making windowframes. Lisa described, and conveyed to me still, her intense pleasure; she said that this had been such fun, and then, rather hurriedly, that it was so nice to do something for Lucinda. Then she hesitated, and I asked her what had happened next. 'Well,' said Lisa unhappily, 'Lucinda went away and left me in the house —I suppose she got bored. She hasn't got much of an attention span—she drifts off out of situations, doesn't she?' I agreed that

[1] *Therapy in Child Care,* ch. 8.

this was so, but added that I felt Lisa was somehow worried about this happening, and asked if this was the case. Lisa at once admitted that she was indeed worried; she felt that she had made some mistake, although she had really helped Lucinda, who could not herself have made window-frames. I suggested that here we might have found the core of the problem; perhaps Lucinda did not like someone else to achieve something beyond her own capacity.

We talked on about this happening, and various points emerged: the most important for Lisa was when she herself realized that what had seemed to her to be kindness and concern for Lucinda was really impingement of a rather awful kind, based on Lisa's wish for an opportunity to take over Lucinda's little house and play in it herself. This realization was reached gradually, working over every detail of the happening. Lisa had been under considerable stress, which was relieved through realization and communication. I was in a position to sympathize with Lucinda (who never did return to the house), and with Lisa, because it is awful to have to recognize ruthlessness and envy operating under cover.

Envy is likely to play quite a part in raising the stress level too high. This same student constantly expressed pity for me, and others: 'You have to work so hard!' or 'It must be awful for you, doing this all the time!' By pitying us she avoided admitting strong and disturbing envy; this eventually emerged in a recognizable form: 'How do you all work like this, without getting fed up and furious? Shall I ever achieve this sort of emotional economy?' This recognition of the envy underlying stress made Lisa's life much easier in the place.

Simple stress can be intolerable (for example, when one has to draw on exhausted emotional reserves when one is very tired); but complex stress, where unconscious envy, hate or guilt is also involved, may be expressed in ways which are destructive both to the worker under stress and to those with whom he comes in contact. Providing the stress can be communicated – the tip of the iceberg, as it were – then there is a good chance (even in complex stress) that the worker will dare to surface the deeper layers, to himself if not to others. In this connection I think it is important to respect the worker's privacy.[1] There *are* people who can contain and deal with a high level of stress within themselves: such people may be children or students. It can be disconcerting if we feel that in the circumstances the person *must* need to communicate stress, and even try to bring this about; when actually this is someone who has a high stress threshold, often because he can tolerate more than the usual amount of insight. We need to be available and accessible to students under stress; but we must leave it to them to choose whether or not to communicate their feelings, unless a point has been reached where the student is actually in reaction to stress, causing harm to others.

Another point which seems important is that the student and the supervisor will both need to be clear that provision of opportunity for communicating stress need not imply subsequent action. Very often, sympathetic and uncritical listening is all that is needed. The sufferer from stress cannot contain his feelings, and needs us to provide containment for the overflow. People often feel that something has got to be *done* at such a moment: I am certain that this is seldom the right time for decisions or actions.

The other danger is the natural wish of the supervisor to replace the often distorted picture presented by the student with the objective reality. This can lead to a logical argument, in the course of which the supervisor can show the student how far from objective reality is his reaction to a situation. However, the point has been missed: the reality which matters in such communication is the reality of the student's feelings–it is with these that the supervisor needs to be concerned, in the management of stress.

There is also the reality of the supervisor's feelings, which cannot be so easily communicated to the student; although, as I have suggested earlier in this paper, it is well worth while making it clear fairly early in the proceedings that we are not omnipotent or omniscient, and that we do not have magical powers which enable us to remain completely calm and undisturbed, in contrast to the rest of humanity. There are, however, problems connected with allowing students to know too much about our feelings.

[1] See ch. 1, p. 11.

I think one could say that one should only communicate enough to enable the student to make allowances for us, in particular circumstances. For example, if one is very worried for personal or professional reasons (or a mixture of the two) it is easy for this to ricochet off and hit the student or anyone else in the environment, without, of course, any intention on one's own part of allowing this to happen. I think it may be advisable in such circumstances to mention to the student, at a suitable moment, that one is in a worried, anxious state for all sorts of reasons; and ask them to bear this in mind if one is irritable or impatient. Otherwise the student, far from accusing one of being bad-tempered and difficult, will be sure that there is something the matter with his work, or that there is something in his personality of which we are showing our disapproval.

One sees this with parents and children: it is well worth while allowing one's children to know that one is worried or in a state about something, and to ask them to bear this in mind if one reacts in all sorts of ways which could be disturbing to them.

This is one of the difficulties of residential supervising, or indeed of residential work of any kind. One is not meeting someone in a session, in an office or consulting room or whatever, for just an hour, in which circumstances one can really be wholly concerned with one's client, although with the departure of the client all our worries will crowd once more into our minds. In residential work, we are coming into contact with other people all the time. The student may need to communicate stress to us just after we have heard that, for example, something has gone wrong with the management of the place, or that a child is in difficulties (perhaps in trouble with the police); and it is extremely difficult, if not impossible, to respond to the student's needs in such a context when we ourselves are under considerable stress. On such occasions I have found it valuable, when I have been deeply involved in residential work myself, to say, 'Of course you can talk to me for a few minutes about what is troubling you, but I may not be much use just now, because I'm worried about several things.' This does imply, of course, an acceptance of the fact that the supervisor is not so very different from the student: just as all residential child care workers have to be able to tolerate the realization that they are not so very different from the children

47

for whom they are caring.

There are other areas where stress may be intolerable, and where communication to the student may present great difficulties. For example, it is possible for the supervisor to feel envy of the student. The student does not have the responsibilities which have to be accepted by the supervisor; the student comes for a short time—the period of the placement—and can then go away, while the supervisor remains to continue his work in the place; the student may have had opportunities which were denied to the supervisor; the very fact that the supervisor tends to be much older than the student can be another reason for experiencing stress complicated by envy. It is perhaps worth considering, whether or not it is desirable for such envy to be communicated to the student: possibly it is quite enough for the supervisor to realize this feeling, or to communicate the stress involved to a colleague; perhaps for this reason supervisors need supervisors! I wonder whether there are many people who can do this kind of work without the opportunity themselves of having some form of safety-valve through communication of stress.

Nobody would willingly get angry with a student or anybody else in a dependent role. Nevertheless, there must be moments when one does feel angry, perhaps due to some insensitivity on the student's part in relation to a disturbed child, or because the student has upset another member of staff or in some way undermined the confidence of a new worker who is just beginning to have some kind of morale in regard to his work in the place. Such a feeling of anger can be difficult to cope with in oneself: as with all types of stress, this feeling can be contained up to a certain level; all that is necessary as a rule is for one to know that one is feeling angry. But the moment many come when it rises above this threshold of toleration: one signal of this can be a physical aspect of anger. It is not for nothing that one talks of somebody going 'white with anger', or 'cold with rage': usually any high degree of stress is accompanied by some physical symptom, which may help one to recognize that one is at that moment beyond one's capacity to contain stress. At such a moment one needs to be extremely careful how one communicates with the student, because it would be terribly easy to be very destructive merely in order to relieve intolerable stress. Perhaps the best thing that one can do in these circumstances is to make a conscious effort to communicate one's concern for the person who has been damaged by the student, rather than one's anger with the student: after all, one's concern will also be a very deep and strong feeling: and after the first flash of anger inside oneself, one may be able to find a way of changing, as it were, one's channel of communication.

The student, on the other hand, may find it very difficult to get angry with us, or rather, the anger will certainly be there, but it will be hard for him to allow this feeling to become conscious, let alone communicable, because of his fears of retaliation. If he is able to get angry with you—in however intolerable a form this may appear, however rude, tiresome and bossy he may be—it is well to remember that the fact that he dares to get angry with you indicates that he trusts you; this is a considerable tribute to you as a person.

It is very easy for both supervisors and students alike to regard the communication of stress as a *symptom*. One can say that all symptoms are actually communications, but this is not to say that the reverse is true (not all communications are symptoms). It is wise to accept that we are all liable to stress; this is not a symptom, nor pathological. Communication can prevent uncontainable stress from turning into a symptom: for example, when one is angry, if one tries to hide the anger one may eventually have a bad headache; the headache *is* a sympton—one no longer feels the anger, which has been converted into the headache.

I feel that supervisors working within residential places with students have an opportunity to help to establish the communication of stress in the students' lives, which can eventually be of great use to both the students and the people with whom they will work later on.

5
Meeting children's emotional needs, 1969

This paper was read to a large Home Office group during a course at Nottingham University in 1969. It brings together a lot of learning experience in a way which led me to further realization. I remember my pleasure and surprise when I met so much sympathy and understanding in my audience (which included senior staff from approved schools). The discussion which followed was of value to me, and the next paper, 'Syndrome', presented during the same course also led to useful communication.

My point of view differs in many ways from that of other disciplines: for example, from that of a teacher. Much that I shall be suggesting may seem irrelevant in the present context of work in residential places: we are in a transitional phase between the publication of the new Act and its implementation. Clearly, there must be development and change—must there also be actual breaks in thought and practice? Are there some ideas or points of view which must be discarded, or can they be adapted to fit a new task?

There is a tendency, because of the close connection between physical and mental health, to think of psychotherapy of any kind as a treatment intended to lead to a cure. Accordingly (for example) the disappearance of specific symptoms in emotional disorder is taken as a sign of recovery; when in fact, the symptom may merely have shifted its ground. Sometimes a behaviour disorder may be replaced by physical symptoms, which will then be treated in the field of physical medicine: this is not a cure. I really wish to jettison the concept of 'cure' at once, and replace this by 'evolvement'. I believe that most people can evolve to some extent, however deeply disturbed they may be, and that in helping our clients to develop emotionally, we ourselves also evolve. There is for me no clear line of demarcation between psychotherapist and patient, teacher and pupil, child care worker and child: we are all *individual people*. Therapy, then, from my own particular viewpoint, involves a relationship between two or more people (individual or group therapy), used in a special and professional way, leading those concerned to further evolvement as unique human beings (Winnicott has pointed out that well people are unique, it is the ill ones who are stereotyped). This realization is essential, especially to those working with deprived and delinquent children. For example, therapeutic work will lead a delinquent to a special kind of depression: it is only too easy to mistake such a manifestation as evidence of deterioration rather than to welcome the onset of a depression as an indication of evolvement without which the delinquent's emotional life must remain static.

I have said that I do not see a clear boundary between workers and clients. Perhaps I should also make clear at this point the fact that I fail to see such a boundary between grownups and children. As I have said before, I regard the word 'adult' as a defence against the realization that we professional people are all *children who have grown up*. There are many parents who tell their children little or nothing about their own childhood: they need to deny the evolvement of the child into the grown-up, and cannot bear their children to think of them in such a way.

It will be realized that I am trying to set up a clear field of communication in which to work. I want my own personal outlook to be understood: it seems important that I should make my position clear. So, I am saying that grown-ups trying to help disturbed children to evolve will *themselves* evolve, provided they can allow relationships to come into existence between grown-ups and children, of which therapeutic use can be made. Just as I am not prepared to think of grown-ups as being other than children grown up, so I am also unwilling to ignore the fact that a sixteen-year-old can have the same needs as the six-months-old, although these needs may be communicated in a distorted, broken down way (we call this 'acting out'). If these needs are not met at six months, or six years or sixteen years or twenty-six years, they will not *change*. The approved schools are having to compensate for the failure of the residential nurseries. One could say of the 'outside' child whom we meet in the approved school, that the shell is made up of defences (to hide the real self) and of broken down communication, taking the form of deviant behaviour. We have to try to understand the nature of the defences, and the communication implicit in the behaviour.

I am advocating a therapy based on *needs* rather than *symptoms*, bearing in mind that many of our clients have been traumatized in one way or another: we are often trying to treat emotionally damaged people who need corrective experience ('corrective' in this sense has no punitive implications). Just what experience may be needed depends on the stage of integration reached by each individual: we need to classify children according to needs based on degree of integration reached. Such classification can be carried out within any kind of residential unit by the people working in the place. If the treatment of the kind I am considering is to become available to the thousands in need of help, then residential units must shoulder the responsibility of providing therapy themselves, rather than looking to outside agencies. This applies equally to residential nurseries and to community homes. Anybody doing residential work with children and young people must learn to make use of therapeutic skills. We have an enormous emotional refugee problem on our hands: thousands of emotionally starved children who are all, in the deepest sense of the word, displaced people. There is nobody beyond us to whom we can hand over this responsibility. Furthermore, a therapy of provision leading to evolvement is not available in a child guidance clinic: such treatment can only be appropriately given in a residential setting, relating as it does to the entire life of the child in need.

It is important that this work should be seen as active, skilled and economic. I am not talking about a permissive environment with minimal controls and structure. There will certainly be no place for corporal punishment or other archaic punitive practices in the new community homes, but it is no use forbidding one kind of management unless it be replaced by another—certainly nothing can evolve in a vacuum. I am, of course, well aware that therapeutic work, such as I have described is being carried out already and I want this to become more conscious and more communicated.

I have spoken of the necessity for classification within a residential unit, based on need and on stage of integration. I must clarify my use of the term 'integration', which is based on Winnicott's concept of integration *as an individual*. I am sure that many of you are accustomed to thinking of integrated or unintegrated children; but, so far, it does not seem usual for residential staff to classify the children in a unit on this basis. When I speak of integration, I am thinking on the lines which Winnicott has postulated.

The populations of residential nurseries, children's homes, and schools for the maladjusted and (up to the present) approved schools, are made up in nearly all cases of a mixture of integrated and unintegrated children. It is essential that the needs of all deprived children should be met: and it must be clearly understood that the nature of these needs depends on degree of integration. So far, it is usual for the behaviour of unintegrated children to be recognized as 'different' from that of others, and to attach labels to them such as behaviour disorders, character disorders, psychopathic personalities, and so on. These labels—technical or otherwise—emphasize the difference between these children and others, while totally failing to suggest that (although they cannot benefit from what is available in the way of management) they are in need of special treatment: this need is so much less easy to recognize, for many reasons, in unintegrated children than in integrated, functioning children, especially because of the breakdown of communication into acting out.

The therapist working with integrated children depends on transference phenomena and on verbal interpretation within the strict limits of the therapeutic hour. The therapist working with unintegrated children must depend on personal involvement, on symbolic actions (adaptations) and on re-establishing communication in place of acting out.

I have worked in two units as a consultant; one catering for five- to twelve-year-olds and specializing in the treatment of severely emotionally deprived unintegrated children who are selected on this basis, and the other an approved school which is still in the difficult phase of change from approved school to therapeutic community. In the first unit (the Mulberry Bush), the only integrated children are those who have evolved to a point at which they are nearly ready to leave the school. In the second (the Cotswold Community) there is at all times a mixture of barely

53

integrated and unintegrated adolescents. It has been possible to classify the approved school children by assessment of integration in the four house groups. This kind of assessment is not usually available in referral reports, but I have found that residential staff are quite able to carry out this sort of in-living diagnosis themselves, in consultation with me. We have used two factors only, in assessing degree of integration: these have been panic and disruption. Where both these factors are present we assume unintegration. Both phenomena are easy to recognize, once their nature is understood. Panic is often described as temper tantrum: disruption as antisocial behaviour. *Panic*, rarely mentioned in psychiatric reports, is the hallmark of unintegration, and represents traumatic—unthinkable—experience at an early age. It produces claustrophobia and agoraphobia, states of disorientation and a total loss of any sense of identity: the victim falls to pieces in a state beyond terror. He may be totally immobilized; or, more frequently, he may hit out, scream, destroy things or attack other people. *Disruption*, described by Erikson as play disruption, can be seen in action very easily. The child comes into a situation where others are functioning, either in work or play, and at once compulsively breaks into the group and breaks up the activity. Panic and disruption are familiar to any experienced worker, but may not have been seen as signals of distress.

It is easier to pick out children who are not integrated, rather than to describe those who are whole, functioning people. My own experience leads me to suppose that in a group of twelve children in residential care—let us say in a children's home—probably two or three will be unintegrated. These children will have an obvious and harmful influence on the lives of the integrated members of the group; while the integrated, functioning children will have very little counter-influence on those who are unintegrated. The mixture of integrated and unintegrated seems to be disastrous for both groups, unless we can find ways of meeting very different needs in the same environment (see chapter 3). I believe this to be possible: whether economic is questionable. On the whole, I feel that there is something to be said for classification to take place as early as possible within the unit, so that living groups can be constituted from similar ingredients, rather than from an explosive mixture of elements.

Within the Cotswold Community there is now a cottage which contains the least integrated group in the community. I think, from what I have seen so far that the cottage group remains therapeutically viable, despite inevitable changes of staff and inmates. On the other hand, each of the eight or nine children in the cottage would cause havoc in other groups: from time to time an unintegrated boy arrives into the community who cannot be placed in the cottage, and one can then see only too clearly how disruptive his presence can be in another group, and how easily he can become either a delinquent hero or a scapegoat. In the same way, any one of the thirty younger children in the Mulberry Bush School would be 'the impossible one' in any normal class, but each becomes manageable in an environment which meets his needs.

I have suggested that a classification of needs can be made, based on two factors–the presence of panic and disruption. Obviously this is a rough-and-ready way to work, and there will always be some borderline cases where it will be difficult to decide the degree of integration. The later the stage of evolvement reached, the less obvious will be the lack of integration. However, nothing can be absolute, and assessment must always be tentative and experimental.

What follows is a scheme or chart, which lists assumptions, aims and techniques, in regard to integrated and unintegrated people of any age, from the standpoint of a psychotherapist. One would say that there must always, in *any* case, be a contract between therapist and patient; a process, whatever needs to to happen between them–evolvement of the patient *and* the therapist.

INTEGRATED	UNINTEGRATED
1. *Assumptions*	
good enough start	not good enough start
identity	projective identification
possibility of transference	no transference, involvement
capacity for guilt	no capacity for guilt
defences, e.g. repression	primitive defences, splitting
boundary between conscious and unconscious	no barrier between conscious and unconscious
symbolization	no symbolization
capacity to contain experiences	

2. *Aims*

sorting out the past	filling gaps in experience
to resolve conflict through transference	to achieve integration as a person
break down crippling defences	through adaptation to reach
enable patient to make full use of potential	regression, containment, with build-up of defences to reach personal guilt, repression, and so on.

3. *Techniques*

use of transference interpretation	involvement with realization symbolic communication adaptation
surfacing of repressed material	

4. *Therapeutic management*

not needed	needed in some or all areas

Very special and long training, including personal analysis, is required to treat integrated patients: in residential work, much that we can achieve for such children depends on our ability to be suitable people with whom children can identify.

We assume that integrated children can identify, having reached secondary experience; but that in the past parental figures have been in some way inadequate: we have to compensate for such inadequacies. The parents will hate and envy us because we are able to help their children in a way which they cannot achieve. We cannot assume that unintegrated children can identify, because they have not reached secondary experience. Here we have to supply missing primary experience, which their deprived parents (or staff in institutions) have been unable to supply. We can expect these parents also to hate us, but they will *envy their children* rather than ourselves, because such parents will know that they themselves have these primary needs (see chapter 2).

Therapeutic work with integrated children in residential treat-

ment is more complex, but less exacting, than work with unintegrated children. Once integrated, children can transfer the deep
confused feelings they have for their parents to us, giving us an
opportunity to understand these feelings, and to help them to
do so, thereby freeing them to identify with us in a new way.
We have to ask ourselves whether we as people can offer them a
better chance to evolve in relation to us and our way of life. It
is not painful to reach understanding of their difficulties, but it
can be very painful to be understood by them—sometimes better
than we understand ourselves.

Unintegrated children present quite other problems. We have
to provide experience which is actually missing from their lives.
They will, in time, accept us with a devastating degree of trust
and dependence. There will be no transference in the ordinary
sense—they cannot transfer what they have not got. They will be
involved with us and we with them in a very simple and primitive
way: our reliability will become our most valuable therapeutic
tool.

Here, then, are the two main groups to be found in all residential work. How much therapy can be carried out in any residential
unit by the people in the place? What is the nature of such therapy?
How can we actually help children to evolve?

Our first task is to produce a suitable emotional climate in the
place, for therapy to be possible. We need to remember that a
therapist, basically, is not a person *doing*, but a person *being*: for
example, people can stop actually punishing but remain punitive.
The right words are no use if they are only a cover for the wrong
feelings. Since child care workers cannot have a personal analysis
and a distinct training as therapists, we need to evolve a mainly
'do-it-yourself' approach, which may help them to gain insight
and free them to become professionally involved with children in
this special way.

People tend to think of therapeutic work as being carried out
in a clinic or consulting room in the course of formal sessions,
over a considerable period of time. Therapy in child care is concerned with the content of the total life situation in the place,
including waking and sleeping, eating and drinking, working
and playing and so on.

To produce the essential emotional climate, if it is not already present, we need to 'clear the decks'. We can most easily make a start in the field of communication, which can become a desert in residential work. There is a tendency to use stereotyped phrases in talking to children, or about them. Workers hide behind these phrases, and the children do likewise: as a result, real feelings are not communicated unless they burst through under stress in the brokendown form which we call 'acting out' (punishment is often acting out). There are various ways of establishing real communication in residential work. You will all be familiar with the writings of David Wills:[1] the concepts of self-government, democratic participation and shared responsibility all involve open and free communication between grown-ups and children; in the course of which, feelings and ideas can be expressed, and respected and used by all. I feel that this sort of approach is ideal for integrated children who have had a good enough start in emotional life, and who are able therefore to experience, realize and conceptualize adequately, in a way which unintegrated children cannot do. Children are encouraged by such work to accept responsibility for being themselves.

At the same time, we must provide them with objects for identification—ourselves. This means in practice a great deal of self-awareness. The worker functioning as a therapist must do so as himself, but with concern, so that he speaks and acts in a responsible and sensitive way in the place. The avoidance of direct and real communication between workers and children aims at preventing the formation of deep personal relationships —which are essential for therapeutic purposes. Therefore, once such communication is established, we can expect these relationships to come spontaneously into existence. When children are integrated, they will transfer to us their conflicts in regard to their parents, and we are then in a position to understand something of their difficulties; and by communicating our understanding, to help them to evolve from long static positions in regard to others.

Institutionalization is a defence against emotional processes: de-institutionalize, and we produce a climate in which these processes can develop *through which people can evolve*. Lack of real

[1] See David Wills, *Throw Away Thy Rod,* Gollancz 1960

communication has a depersonalizing effect, and the establishment–or re-establishment–of communication is an essential
first measure to make therapeutic work possible.

It is a much easier task to establish communication with integrated children than with unintegrated ones. The latter group
must be considered carefully because this is the source of most
problems in any residential work. I have already mentioned the
tendency of unintegrated children to panic and to disrupt the
functioning of others. I have found that small groups of four
children and one grown-up, meeting each morning for about
half an hour, can eventually reach intercommunication. Such
a group can be mixed in degree of integration (a ratio of one
unintegrated to three integrated), but ideally *not* mixed, so that
the functioning of the integrated does not threaten the unintegrated. The beginning of such work will probably be extremely
discouraging, but communication will come with patience and
empathy.

In order to understand the therapeutic value of invariable
response to all communication from children of any age, it is
important to grasp the concept of 'the spontaneous gesture'
(Winnicott). The baby smiles at the mother and reaches out to
her: the mother's response is an essential to the baby's emotional
wellbeing. If the mother does not or cannot (because of her own
defences) respond to the spontaneous gesture, then the baby
is reaching out as though for ever into infinity. Eventually in
such a case the baby ceases to attempt those gestures, having
reached despair. Our response to what a deprived child tries to
communicate may re-establish his belief in the possibility of response to his reaching out. Recently a child aged ten called Timothy
drew for me a picture of himself in his cot as a baby: the picture
showed him lying flat in the cot with one hand showing between
the bars. He said, 'That's me trying to reach my mum–it's a bit
like a cage, the cot, isn't it?' I replied that this was so, but that
perhaps the bars of this cage also kept his mother away from him
–were also the bars of *her* cage: in other words, her defences,
protecting him from her violence, but also isolating him.

We have to be careful that children find *us* when they reach
out, and that they do not again find defences instead of people.
A boy at the Cotswold Community said to me: 'It's different

here from the other place.' I asked what was the greatest difference, to which he answered: 'People really listen to you—they don't just hear you—they *listen*—nobody has ever listened to me like that before.'

Sometimes people are afraid of what children will say, of the dreadful unanswerable questions they may ask: this is a valid fear, but it is also valid to say that just listening is therapy. At first much that our clients will say will be paranoid accusations and complaints against all who are in authority of any kind, complaints without logical reasoning. We can listen to such complaints, accepting the reality of the feelings expressed and leaving the objective reality alone for the present. Gradually the child will start to communicate his dread and his helplessness.

We are, I assume, considering the whole range of residential displacement, residential nurseries, children's homes, schools for maladjusted children, and approved schools. In all these institutions I suspect that there is a larger proportion of unintegrated children than is realized—this is not a policy, but a relatively unconsidered fact.

Let us now take a look at the needs of these unintegrated children. With integrated neurotic children, we can assume the presence of an identity, a functioning ego, a capacity for concern (personal guilt), and anxiety (repressed guilt). None of these assumptions hold good when we come to consider those who have not achieved the establishment of identity. We are now considering the terribly deprived ones—those whose needs have not been met during the first year of life. I have elsewhere described[1] the syndromes which develop in terms of the nature of the traumatic interruption of emotional development and the point at which this has taken place. Here I must quote my descriptions of these syndromes of deprivation.

The most primitive of these categories, that is to say the least integrated, is made up of those whom I have described elsewhere as the 'frozen' children; who have suffered interruption of primary experience at the point where they and their mothers

[1] *Therapy in Child Care*, ch. 9, 'The provision of primary experience in a therapeutic school'.

[1] *Ibid.*, p. 99.

would be commencing the separating out process, having been as it were broken off rather than separated out from their mothers. They have survived by perpetuating a pseudosymbiotic state; without boundaries to personality, merged with their environment, and unable to make any real object relationships or to feel the need for them.

Such a child must be provided with the actual emotional experiences of progression to separating out; thereby establishing identity, accepting boundaries, and finally reaching a state of dependence on the therapist. This kind of child cannot symbolize what he has never experienced or realized. (A 'frozen' child, on referral, will steal food from the larder because he wants food at that moment and for no other reason. The same child in the course of recovery may steal again from the larder, because his therapist is absent; this stealing will now be symbolic.)

The next category consists of those who have achieved the first steps towards integration; so that one could describe them as made up of ego-islets which have never fused into a continent—a total person. For this reason we call them 'archipelago' children. These children give the impression of being quite mad whenever they are not being quite sane. They are either wildly aggressive, destructive, and out of touch in states of panic-rage or terror; or they are gentle, dependent, and concerned. They present a bewildering picture till one comes to know them and to understand the meaning of their behaviour. They too need to progress through the process of integration. However, these stormy children are not so difficult to help as 'frozen' children, because the presence of ego-islets amid the chaos of unassimilated experience makes life more difficult for them. They are, from time to time, very unhappy and aware that they need help. The fact that some primary experiences have been contained and realized results in their having a limited capacity for symbolization, which facilitates communication of a symbolic kind which is not available to 'frozen' ones. Where 'frozen' and 'archipelago' children are concerned, treatment must involve the breakdown of pathological defences, containment of the total child, and the achievement of dependence on the therapist as a separate person. These two groups, in which integration has not been sufficient to establish a position from which to regress, are very different from those in the next category.

Classifying the 'false-self' organizations, Winnicott writes: 'At one extreme: the false-self sets up as real and it is this that

Consultation in child care

observers tend to think is the real person. In living relationships, work relationships, and friendships, however, the false-self begins to fail. In situations in which what is expected is a whole person the false-self has some essential lacking. At this extreme the true-self is hidden.' Having described other types of false-selves advancing towards health, he continues: 'Still further towards health: the false-self is built on identifications (as for example that of the patient mentioned whose childhood environment and whose actual nannie gave much colour to the false-self organization).'

The latter organization he has described as the 'caretaker-self'. This elaborate defence takes various forms, and is often difficult to recognize, especially because the 'little self' part of the child is carefully concealed by the caretaker (for example, there may be a delinquent 'caretaker' which steals without conflict, on behalf of the 'little-self').

Therapeutic work with these deeply deprived children involves one in making adaptations to their needs, much as the 'ordinary devoted mother' (Winnicott) makes adaptations to the needs of her babies. It is important to realize at once that there is nothing impossible about this task, which is being carried out constantly in therapeutic institutions. The easiest approach is to introduce certain adaptations oneself, which become 'part of life'. As I have said before, all children should have hotwater bottles, a special drink, and the chance to communicate when they are in bed, before they go to sleep. Such provision will soon become highly individual. A child will choose a bottle of this colour, will write his name on it, will need it filled so full and so hot, and for the bottle to be placed in his bed, or given to him, or whatever. You can see how depersonalization can be tackled by such means. Provision like this can be made either based on an individual relationship established between child and grown-up, or between the child and the house team. In any event there must be constant communication between members of the treatment team, so that everybody becomes aware of the individual needs of each child. While it is always difficult to embark on provision, the rewards are so instant that the work becomes easier as staff gain confidence.

Food is an area of provision which is all too often utterly institutionalized. Delinquent excitement is frequently a displacement from frustrated infantile greed. Food available when needed can often help to bring this excitement back into the oral zone where it belongs. There must be plenty of milk and snacks available on request (as Derek Miller found):[1] but the food, in my view, should always *be given by somebody*, rather than be collected by the child from the larder.

Society tends to be punitive in regard to food in institutions: not enough money is assigned to food in the budget; cooking is impersonal, in bulk, and frequently unappetising. Ideally each group should be eating in the unit or cottage, rather than with the whole population in one large dining hall. It is interesting to note that meals eaten in small groups take much longer than those *en masse*, because the children talk and enjoy themselves personally over a meal in their own group, whereas they eat their food and go as soon as possible when eating in a dining hall.

Children in rigid institutions are constantly exposed to further frustration and deprivation, which lead, of course, to subcultures and depravity—for which they are punished, thus creating a vicious circle.

Many people in child care would spontaneously work in the way I have described: they often only need permission, encouragement and support to become therapists. Very often in a rigid institution such workers may be criticized, discouraged and undermined: this is true in every field—in hospitals, schools, and children's homes. Leadership roles in a therapeutic community must be distinct and reliable. The 'director' (or whatever he may be termed), the head of group living, the head of each unit, or the housemother, must be linked by principles and free communication on a basis of mutual support. Women need to be able to work professionally and in role, not confining their activities to mending and housework. A group of men and women working together as therapists, helping each other to understand the problems of the children in their care, can achieve a high standard of therapeutic skill. They will need to read, and to talk over and apply what they read to their experience, in order to learn how to add therapeutic attitudes to their various skills and to accept roles within their specific functions as teachers, craftsmen or houseparents.

I was involved in a very interesting and valuable experience

[1] See Derek Miller, *Growth to Freedom,* Tavistock 1964, pp. 109 and 178.

which took place between a carpentry instructor and a deprived delinquent boy. Tommy had become interested in chess and the history of the game. He could play very well, and he decided that he wished to make his own chess set. He was interested in an eighteenth century chess set which I had been given, and I brought a piece to show him. He was fascinated by the survival of the set, and wondered about the craftsmen who had carved the pieces with such skill, so long ago. He suggested that if he now made a chess set, this might also survive into some future century, and in any case he could hand the set down to his son. This was the first time I had heard Tommy talking about any distant future or past (like most delinquents, he lived in the present exclusively). I explained about Tommy's wish to the carpentry instructor, who gave him the considerable amount of help and support that he needed to carve the queen, which he brought to show me on my next visit. Subsequently he carved the king, and then a remarkably fat pawn (he is a solid little person himself). Tommy was delighted by his achievement, and we all eagerly awaited further developments.... There were none. Tommy was satisfied by what to him was a complete experience. He had symbolized a family – a father, a mother and one child, which was what he would have wished his family to be. A chess set became irrelevant in terms of his symbolization. Nobody urged him to continue a task which, however incomplete for us, was finished for him: he values his three pieces highly, and so do we all. Here is an example of therapeutic work action within the normal structure of a residential place.

I have written a paper on the subject of therapeutic play in residential work:[1] I find it difficult to condense such a large subject into any sort of summary. I have suggested that – in common with other therapeutic measures – therapeutic play depends on the provision of a suitable emotional climate. Everyone is ready to teach children how to play games: therapeutic play comes from inside the children themselves, many of whom have never played in this symbolic way. There is, however, no need to interpret this sort of play – to tease out the meaning of the children's use of play material: interpretation of play belongs to play therapy, whereas opportunities for therapeutic play can be provided by

---

[1] See 'Play as therapy in child care' *Therapy in Child Care,* ch. 11

workers in residential places of all kinds, and for children of all ages.

You will realize from what I have said that here again, the play groups need to be classified into integrated and unintegrated, with never more than eight children in a group, with one therapist-worker.

There will always be occasional children who need more intensive treatment–psychotherapy or even hospitalization. Such decisions can only be reached on the advice of a consultant psychiatrist. It would seem that there will be intensive care units for very ill children who need to be insulated and contained for treatment to be possible. Most children, however, could be treated within the proposed framework of a community home, where (presumably) a child guidance team will be available to the whole community. I would hope that some of the work of such a team would be available for use in the further training of staff, through lectures, films and discussion groups.

At first any consultant will be felt as a threat to the people in the place; then, probably, in the next phase as some sort of magical messiah 'who knows all the answers'. Eventually, however, there is a good chance that the consultant will be reasonably in role, working in a structured and carefully planned way, known to all and used economically and to further primary tasks (i.e. not regarded as a resource for the grown ups, to the exclusion of the children).

As a consultant psychotherapist I work in the two units already mentioned on much these lines. Most of my work takes the form of group discussions: at the Mulberry Bush I also meet the child care staff as a group, and I have an individual session with each member of the team every week. I see children 'on demand' for short or long sessions, and I meet the headmaster weekly. All these meetings are based on whatever people wish to discuss with me, with the exception of one weekly meeting with the whole team (about fifteen people), when we consider a context profile which has been built up by everyone, including myself. This kind of reporting in depth seems to have special values in residential work. In order to make a context profile, the team choose a child for special consideration, and then report on all their experiences (not observations) with this child in the course of a week. At the end of a week, during which I have a session with the child, we meet to pool experiences, and discuss the implications in terms of the child's own needs, and how these can be met at this point. This is an oversimplified description: 'Context profiles' is a paper in *Therapy in child care*.

SUMMARY

I must apoligize for the fact that I have as it were painted a picture, instead of producing a blue-print for therapy in residential work. I hope, however, that I have succeeded in showing you, what many of you must already know, that therapy belongs within the context of everyday life in a place. There can be no therapeutic work without the foundation of relationships between grown-ups and children: you cannot do therapy in an emotional vacuum, however precise the dosage.

There must be *communication*—real, uncensored communication, which means that grown-ups at all levels have to listen in a very special way to anything which children say, however apparently rude or irrelevant. There must also be this real communication between the grown-ups themselves, who can then pool their resources. There will be adaptation to individual needs in groups—provision of primary and transitional experience among un-integrated children, and opportunites and support for functioning among integrated children. For this to be possible there must be classification according to integration, and assessment and re-assessment of stage of integration reached. There is a need for consultation to be available to grown-ups and children, individually and in groups.

But above all, therapy needs to be seen as a recognition of needs—deep, urgent needs—which must be met with concern.

6
Syndrome, 1970

I have already mentioned (p. 50) that this paper was read during a Home Office course at Nottingham University in 1969. My intention is to write other 'syndromes' describing all the syndromes of deprivation (described in 'The Provision of primary experience', 'Therapy in Child Care, ch.9).

I am going to try in this paper to describe a syndrome of deprivation–what Winnicott calls 'caretaker self'. I described this syndrome briefly in Chapter 5.

I want to convey to you the *feeling* of this syndrome; how it appears in a baby in a residential nursery, in a child in a children's home, a school for maladjusted children, and finally in an approved school. All my descriptions will be real, in that they will be based on actual clinical material about severely emotionally deprived children at different ages. Ideally, I should be giving the whole history of one such child, but I have never had the opportunity of tracing such an individual from babyhood to adolescence. What I have actually done, therefore, is to build the early history on case material and clinical descriptions of deprivations in early childhood. Subsequently, I shall be able to quote from personal experience with actual 'caretaker-selves' at later stages in residential places and from discussion with people working with them.

What is so striking about any syndrome of deprivation is the lack of change in the child (or indeed, adolescent or grown-up). Their defences remain as established in babyhood, until their needs are met–when at last they can begin to grow emotionally.

My first piece of clinical material will describe the formation of the caretaker-self syndrome during the first year of the life of a baby whom I shall call James. James was an illegitimate child: his mother was a girl of sixteen, herself deprived and delinquent. We know nothing about his father, and practically nothing concerning his mother, who handed James over for adoption and disappeared for ever from his life, when he was about three weeks old. His actual birth was prolonged and traumatic, and he was a delicate baby. He was adopted by a couple, Mr and Mrs B, who were devoted to him. Mrs B was capable of the deep maternal preoccupation without which he probably would not have survived: because of the following months in Mrs B's care, James gained enough primary experience to build an ego—a self, fragile and delicate like a young plant, but established through her love and reliability.

When James was about nine months old, Mrs B died as the result of a sudden illness. Mr B was inconsolable. His own parents and those of Mrs B were very involved with the baby; they introduced into the house a nurse-housekeeper, to take charge of James under their guidance, and to run the house for Mr B. This housekeeper, Mrs Smith, was a cold, efficient person. She took every care of James from a physical point of view, but was rigid and punitive in her management of him, so that he was deprived of maternal love, and was looked after in an institutionalized way. Mr B was so sunk in mourning for his wife that he put all his energy into his business. When at home, however, he was kind and concerned about James—but too exhausted and unhappy to realize how emotionally ill James was becoming. The grandparents on both sides approved of Mrs Smith's care of James: but from the first they over-indulged and stimulated him in a way which had nothing to do with the baby's needs—but everything to do with their own. There was rivalry between both pairs of grandparents, and a sort of possessiveness in regard to James, but more as a thing than a person.

As I have said, James had been able to establish a fragile ego from the good experience given to him by his adoptive mother. Now he was no longer picked up and held when he cried; and he was fed on a rigid schedule, not when he was hungry. At first he was inconsolable: he cried incessantly, refused food, had constant digestive upsets, and slept very badly. It was noticed that he put his thumbs under his armpits, apparently trying to raise himself: I think that at this point (aged ten months) he was trying to *be* the mother who used to lift him up in her arms. Because he now often had to wait too long for his feeds, he would become desperately excited and greedy, but eventually lose the excitement and greed; so that by the time Mrs Smith brought his feed, he was not excited any more, though he accepted the feed. Presently the excitement became split off from food and was felt in other contexts (eventually this orgiastic excitement went into the field of delinquency).

James became apparently completely accepting of the rigid regime imposed by Mrs Smith. He was habit trained early, was clean and 'good', rarely cried, but continued to sleep very little. He responded to stimulation with apparent delight, but he did nothing spontaneous. He *returned* smiles, but he did not initiate any communication. Somehow he managed to maintain a sort of inner reality. He himself became the mother who looked after her baby–his real self. The 'mother' part of him, however, became modelled on the pattern of Mrs Smith. One could say that the harsh introjected super-ego of Mrs Smith took over the care of the fragile ego-id which was James himself. He became extremely reserved, inhibited and secret, hiding his real self in order to insure his survival. He became in effect *two* people: James the stern nurse guarding his charge, and James the instinctual, frantic and excited baby – hidden for the most part, but always present within him.

From time to time the defence–the caretaker–broke down, and James would become very ill, running high temperatures: these illnesses puzzled the family doctor. One day it would be the instinctual, excited little self which would break away into delinquency, but this was years later. We leave James at eighteen months.

Peter was the third and youngest child of a fairly united marriage. His elder brother and sister were aged eight and nine when he was born, so that in a way he was rather like an only child. He was unplanned, but not unwanted, nevertheless his arrival on the scene presented problems. Both his parents were working, and his mother, Mrs M, had become used to the professional life to which she had returned when the older children started school. Mrs M, like Mrs B, was capable of maternal preoccupation with her babies. This tie proved stronger than her wish to return to work for the first few months of Peter's life (his birth was normal). For various reasons Mrs M's unmarried sister lived with the family at this time, and once Peter was weaned, Mrs M arranged with

her sister–Miss C–that she should take over the care of Peter.
who had, up to this point, been a normal and happy baby. Mr M
was glad that this was possible, because Mrs M's earnings made a
considerable difference to the family income. Mrs M was only
devoted to her babies for the first months of their lives. This plan
need not have been disastrous had the sister, Miss C, been a
maternal person who could have to some extent represented his
mother, providing transitional experience which could have
prevented deprivation. As it was, the long periods which Peter
spent in the care of Miss C became for the most part gaps in emotional experience–gaps, because they were unthinkable. These
histories of severe deprivation all stem from a pre-verbal period,
so that only pre-verbal communication is available: babies cannot
think about their troubles, only *feel* them.

Peter spent long periods sitting silent and 'well behaved' in
his cot or pram: his world, seen in this way, remained two-di-
mensional. He had no opportunities to discover the depth of his
environment through tactile experience. This perceptual problem
was later to result in disorientation and severe panic states (these
were really states of helpless rage). I want you to imagine Peter,
at the age of eighteen months and about two feet high, standing
at the top of a staircase. The stairs from his viewpoint would
appear as a smooth precipice. Normally he would have discovered
the steps by sitting with his mother and bumping gently down
them. Peter was deprived of such experience, so that he became
terrified of stairs. Perhaps his aunt, Miss C, *explained* to him about
the nature of a staircase, but this was no use to him at all. This is
the mistake that so many people make–to suppose that conceptualization can precede experience. This is only one example of
failure in adaptation.

Miss C left Peter's home when he was just two years old. The
damage was already done; Peter was a conforming, grave little
boy, always quiet, polite and obedient. He ate little, slept badly
and was beginning to have severe attacks of panic, which were
seen as temper tantrums. He also had physical breakdowns into
respiratory illness. His mother felt that he was now her sister's
child: because of lifelong problems between them, she unconsciously rejected Peter, who now seemed so like her sister, Miss C.

Peter's mother suddenly became ill and was hospitalized. The older children went to stay with their grandmother in the country. Peter, on the advice of the family doctor, was placed in a small residential nursery near his home. Those of you who have seen the latest Robertson film 'John' will have some idea of the dangers implicit in such a placement. John, however, was a normal integrated little boy when he entered the nursery: Peter was already so damaged that this placement only strengthened the pathological defence. The workers in the nursery found him cooperative and quiet. Nobody thought of him as a seriously ill little boy: nobody saw his so *very* good and prim behaviour as evidence of deep deprivation. They noticed that he preferred to stay in one place, that he did not eat much, and was not physically strong. One worker described him as 'old-fashioned'. Most of the other small children in the nursery had been institutionalized for some time. They rushed about, were excited and aggressive, communicated in an institutionalized way, and tended to attack Peter. The workers were unfailingly kind, and physical standards were excellent, but they had no insight into the problems of deprivation; and the terrible shift system (*still* in existence) made any continuity of care by one person impossible.

By the end of the months which Peter had spent in the nursery — although he was visited by his father — he was doomed. He was not to find the primary experience he needed until he was fifteen years old. Until then, nobody except Peter himself knew of the existence of his real self. He led a narrow, restricted life, interrupted by illness and panic states, until his breakdown in adolescence.

Very little could be established about Richard's early life because his mother was terribly vague and unreliable. His father had left when Richard was a baby: he was taken into care when he was about two years old and was placed in a foster home. Mrs V, his foster mother, loved him deeply, and from various bits of evidence it seems that he must have had a much needed regression to a babyhood state in this home. By this, I mean the organized regression of which Winnicott writes; in which the patient returns to that point at which maternal adaptation failed, and receives in actual or symbolic form the kind of care which is needed by babies, thereby filling the gaps in emotional experience which are always to be found in cases of emotional deprivation. Five years later, Richard could convey to me the warmth and security which he felt during this period with Mrs V.

This was not to last. Mrs V and her husband wished to adopt Richard – but at this point Richard's mother suddenly demanded that he should be returned to her. Unimaginably, Richard was dragged away from a despairing Mrs V. He said to me later: 'They must have known – we both cried and cried.' The Vs left the district. Richard meanwhile struggled miserably with his own family. He could not talk about Mrs V at home: he tried not to lose all that she meant to him, whilst keeping his love – and his despair – secret. He developed the symptom of soiling, which was in fact symbolic communication of his inability to keep the secret of his hidden need for Mrs V. His mother rejected him and was so punitive towards him that he was again taken into care (at her request), and established in a children's home at the age of five years.

Here he continued to soil, and to keep his real self (the baby who had had a start with Mrs V) hidden from everybody. Apart from the soiling symptom, Richard was not a difficult child to manage, although the staff in the home found him cold and reserved.

In this case we can see the formation of the caretaker–self syndrome at a much later stage of development. One can assume that Richard had a very bad start with massive deprivation during the first year. By the time he reached Mrs V, he was probably as institutionalized, cold and violent as the toddlers in the film of 'John'.[1] He would probably have emerged as a 'frozen' delinquent, but Mrs V's provision brought about a change in direction: Richard had a therapeutic breakdown in her care which strengthened his embryonic ego. The traumatic separation from her resulted in the caretaker (the Richard who was rigid, cold and reserved) and the 'secret' little self, built from the experience with Mrs V, but of necessity hidden from his jealous and rejecting mother, and subsequently from everyone. Much later, when I met him in treatment in a therapeutic school, I asked, 'But Richard, why have you never talked about this before to anyone?' He replied: 'There was never anyone to talk *to* – nobody who would

---

[1] *Young children in brief separation, no. 3, John,* James and Joyce Robertson, Tavistock Child Development Research Unit 1969

understand.' He was very grateful to the psychiatrist who had recognized the severity of his illness and had secured treatment for him. He has now had a further regression, and is beginning to evolve.

I have spoken about 'context profiles'. I am now going to quote from a Mulberry Bush profile at some length, because this profile concerns another child called Joseph at the age of eleven; in the course of treatment in a therapeutic school he has evolved from a devastating, frozen delinquent to a caretaker-self syndrome, and in such a conscious way that he has been able to report on the process. We have often had referrals who have turned out to be 'caretakers', but this is the first time that we have been able to recognize the formation of the syndrome as it was happening, at such a late age.

My description of a frozen child in Chapter 9 of *Therapy in Child Care* is quoted on p. 99.

One such child was Joseph. At one time we really wondered whether we could continue to contain Joseph in the Mulberry Bush. It seemed to us, at the end of two years' work, that no basic evolvement was taking place, despite carefully planned provision of primary experience by the treatment team. A description of Joseph on referral *still* seemed only too valid at this point. After much discussion, however, we decided to struggle on for a little longer, knowing that if nothing could be achieved, he would certainly become a criminal.

The first sign that I could see of change was Joseph's initial use of symbols. He came to see me, and in the course of a session he communicated for the first time in a symbolic way. A little later it became clear that he was now capable of experiencing a sense of personal guilt, and as one would expect, this achievement brought with it the possibility of depression, and dependence of an early kind.

He came one day for a session. We played 'squiggles' together as usual. I had written his name in full at the top of the first piece of paper: under this he wrote 'JO' within a circle, carefully drawn. This was the first intimation of the presence of his little self—not that I recognized this at the time.

Joseph began gradually to talk of Jo. He told me that little Jo was the size of his thumb, that he constantly was trying to escape and get into mischief, that Joseph had to keep a firm hold on little Jo's hand, because he would run away. He said: 'Jo has to be fed an awful lot, and he needs a long time in the bath. I must always know where he is. He ran away once when he had the nightmare. He's a day older than me—that's how he knew I'd be born. That's how he looked out into the future. He looked out ahead of life. He knew what was coming but he didn't tell me. I'd have been scared, wouldn't I...? Jo had a dream once about ghosts—the ghost chased him out of my bedroom, so for one minute he wasn't with me, so he almost died of horror. We need each other.'

On another occasion, Joseph was riding on Roger Matthew's back.

R.M.   You talked about teeth again.
J.   Yes (it's the same).
R.M.   The time before was in your bedroom.
J.   That was when the room exploded.
R.M.   Because your vest wasn't folded the right way.
J.   *(Tape not clear at this point).*
R.M.   When the vest was folded neatly it was alright.
J.   When it wasn't folded—that was bad—that was the wrong way.
R.M.   It was crumpled and mixed up.
J.   That was the bad way, that's why the room would explode.
R.M.   Does it work just with your vest?
J.   It's just this vest I've got on, it's a magic vest. *(Pulls it out.)*
R.M.   I see.
J.   It's just this vest, it's a bit broken.

We discussed this material about Joseph's vest in a context profile. There was a great deal of discussion in the course of this profile, so I have only time to select a few passages from it.

Myself: I am awfully interested about the vest. I've thought and thought about it because it's turned up other times and I've come to the conclusion that the vest is Joseph's description of Freud's barrier against stimuli; his whole way in which he describes the vest suggests that the vest is a protection from impingement: you notice it is so important that it's folded in the right way, and he says 'It's a magic vest' and 'It's a bit broken.' And one would assume from this bit 'It's a bit broken' that this means he has not got something sufficiently protective between him and the outside world; this is not defence in the ordinary sense—a barrier against stimuli is something that Freud described as being provided by the mother and by the environment to protect the baby from impingement—he didn't put it quite like that, but he *did* talk about a barrier against stimuli, and that if this is broken through then there is a lack of a normal protective area, which is actually needed. This comes in very much with frozen children: they simply haven't got a barrier against stimuli, they merge, they haven't got an edge to themselves; they haven't got this barrier which separates them from outside —invasion, impingements, attack, breaking-in—however you like to think of it; and Joseph's use of the vest and the way he speaks about the vest suggests this to me—it's a rather interesting piece of description, the feeling that there is something of this sort that he knows he needs and hasn't really got, so he has a magic vest: but it's broken, it's not really adequate, it doesn't really work—and I am sure it doesn't.

John Armstrong: I am sure that this vest is significant for him; nevertheless, vests are not things that he looks after: he will treat a vest as he treats all his other clothes—he will throw them about. In addition to this it would be interesting to know, if this is so, what sort of climate he was experiencing when he spent so much time getting rid of this vest and not wearing it, when he should be wearing it.

Myself: Well, this would absolutely fit (I didn't know this about Joseph and his vest), in that frozen children don't want such a barrier. When they are really at their illest they want no barrier, they want nothing that prevents them merging with the environment: their aim is re-establishing symbiosis; so, of course, they are not looking for a barrier against stimuli, they use merger instead, in which there is no question of boundaries, or edges or barriers of any kind, and they are terrified by barriers, and panic when barriers are imposed—in other words what we would call imposing boundaries, on such a person, produces panic for this reason.

Douglas Hawkins: Would the vest be symbolic, then?

Myself: Yes. I was simply thinking that he is using this as a symbolic realization, of which he is perfectly capable: I know, because of other material he's produced, and one would be expecting him to achieve symbolization at this point: there's plenty of it in this material, and there's plenty of it in lots of other material which he is producing now; and at this stage one would expect symbolization. In fact this road is well charted, isn't it? One can look out for things and hope to find them at certain stages: it is usually a question of whether one is in a position to see them or not—whether they do become apparent or not. This is not just Joseph, this is any such child at such a stage. It could be anything in Joseph's case; at the moment it is chance, I think, that he chooses the vest for this piece of description, but it is next to his skin, and so when it's not there it *is* there, is my guess now—you know, that he feels there is a vest next to his skin, he feels there's something, there is a protective barrier that is between him and the outside, that he has got a container, there is something that contains him—and he's got an inside and an outside.

D.H. Is this something that's growing?

Myself: Yes, that's right, and consciousness of the existence of Jo, for example, would make this very distinct: the outside world would be looking after the inside.

SECOND EXTRACT

J.A. More and more, I think there's good value for us in continuing this discussion.

Myself: Well, he represents such a lot, doesn't he? He's a very representative person and he's in a process, so that—in a sense—one is able to see what's happening. I've discussed him from time to time with various people who have been working with him, so I've heard a lot about Joseph.

J.A. We really didn't get much past the 'Last Will and Testament' and there is a great deal besides that.

Myself: I've got my own notes on a session I had with Joseph and I would like to discuss these at some point.

R.M. I think I discussed this with you once—in Brian's room there is a chest of drawers and one drawer has been taken out—

Myself: Of course! I remember.

R.M. —and he said 'This is like a mouth', and I didn't understand that, so I let him go on, and I finally realized that it was like a

76

row of teeth with one missing: he then went on to ask me about whether teeth grew again, and I said that only one set of teeth grow again, and that they don't carry on growing.

J.A. Was this recently?

Myself: No, quite a time back, but we had forgotten about it.

R.M. About three weeks after I came.

Myself: I remember clearly, you telling me about it, and how interesting it was because one could see just how he would feel: it looks so like a hole, where a drawer is taken out of a chest of drawers.

R.M. This is a little drawer, as well.

Myself: Yes. You know, one could so easily say 'Well, aren't these castration anxieties?' but my own feeling is that this isn't about this at all, but it is something much more basic and much more to do with the self and identity, and gaps, and all this; so that one could make a mistake...except, that, of course, it could be things at two levels. Could I discuss the notes on my session with Joseph at this point? It wasn't, in a way, a very valuable session for me, but there was very interesting material in it all the same. This was his first squiggle, what he made of it, he said was a house. I said, 'Whose?' and he said, 'Mine'. *Me:* 'What do you do in it?' *Joseph:* 'I stay up to midnight, two nights a week.' *Me:* 'What about the lines all over the house?' *Joseph:* 'The lines are the bricks.' (Then Joseph sort of stopped.) *Me:* 'What do you do in the house?' *Joseph:* 'I play all sorts of games – Lotto, and things like that.' He then drifted off and there wasn't really very much to it. This is the second squiggle, and Joseph said, 'It is a pattern of a star, it reminds me of Apollo 8...9...10.' *Me:* 'Could that be three years of your life?' *Joseph:* 'Ummm . .' *Me:* 'You've been some pretty big journeys in the last three years.' (Really, I was thinking of when he talked about the stages and the phases, earlier.) *Joseph:* 'I've been to Paddington and I've been to . . .' He took this up at a reality level. I didn't want to drift off into this sort of thing, so I asked whether Jo also went on journeys to Paddington and things like that. Joseph has spoken of Jo to me quite often, so this was appropriate. *Joseph:* 'He went to the seaside without me when I was asleep at night: he's always going. In the daytime he climbs trees, sometimes with me, and sometimes without; he always goes on walks with me, I always hold his hand in case he runs away, and of course he sleeps with me. He was ten on Christmas day.' I rather missed out on this one because this would be Jesus, presumably, and Jo... and all sorts of associations ... could be.

J.A. You know that this is Joseph's birthday?

Myself: Oh no, I didn't know anything of the sort. Well, this explains that one–I had forgotten all about Christmas Day being his birthday: this couldn't be simpler, this being the case. Then this was the third squiggle. *Joseph:* 'A fat person: that's what Jo looks like with his disguise, but much smaller, he's only so big in real life' (indicating with his thumb). Here again, I thought this could so easily be a reference to his penis–his thumb and little Jo could be his penis, and this is not at all unusual, and could be the kind of thing that would turn up. Then I thought something that I had not really thought clearly before: when you get symbolization taking place, the last thing one wants to do is to interpret it, because one is only setting the child back to where he was before he symbolized; there's no reason to interpret, it is the last thing you'd think of doing. And, really, I thought it quite probable that the penis represents Jo, rather than that Jo represents the penis.

J.A. Yes, and this made me suddenly think of Julian and his little bear stuck down the front of his trousers.

Myself: Yes, exactly. One could make a great mistake by seeing this the wrong way round; that it really matters an awful lot which way round it is, and one would have to think awfully carefully and watch the material that emerged about this. I was thinking about other material which could point in the same direction, which was why I was thinking about this business of castration fears and so on, and why I was saying it needn't be castration fears, it could be fears for little Jo, who could be represented by his penis, but the basis is there for identity, and himself. And this is where, I think, a lot of people go frightfully wrong.... I'm still a bit confused about it myself, but I think it makes sense. Then Joseph went on: 'Connie still gives me money–half for Jo and half for me.'

J.A. Usually it's two sixpences.

Myself: Well, there you are, and it absolutely fits the material.

Joseph said, 'Same with dinner . . . I bet he won't like the pudding and I'll have to eat both.' This struck me as in a way terribly funny, because of the obvious complications of such a situation – and he went on to say how much Jo likes custard and he doesn't – so Jo can have all the custard. The amount of planning that must go into this! Then Joseph said of Jo, 'He ate my sleeve and made a big hole in it.' Now, isn't there a hole in the vest? I rather wondered whether this was Jo from inside or impingement from outside, or a mixture of both – I just couldn't decide. Joseph, continuing, said '. . . . and my trousers, he makes holes in my blankets and sheets.' *Me:* 'It sounds as though he needs to bite a lot.' *Joseph:* 'Yes, *he does.* I used to hit him a lot, I don't now, I hardly ever hit him now.' That's the lot. It's interesting, isn't it?

THIRD EXTRACT

J.A. I was just thinking, upstairs there must be some forty-five records, and there is only one without a centre, and this is Joseph's, and it's the only record he has, as far as I know. I put it on last and it's quite a job because it doesn't sit on to the thing and you have to get it just right or it goes into orbit, and, of course, it *would* be Joseph's. *He* didn't make an enlarged hole, he did a swop with somebody for it and it had this hole before he came by it.

Myself: Really, it's extraordinary, isn't it? They link up so relevantly, don't they? I was thinking about the hole, and his mouth and the teeth, and Jo, and the possibility of something Winnicott described a long time ago about a child who had emotionally lost his mouth, and we discussed this in terms of a deprived child: at that time, he ate and spoke and so on, but in fact he didn't feel as though he had got a mouth.

J.A. It might as well have been a tube, or something.

Myself: That's right. It had to do with his mother's breast, that there had to be a breast for him to have a mouth, and that is what had been missing – there hadn't been the breast for his mouth, so the mouth didn't come alive.

J.A. Well, there was no demand for it, was there?

Myself: One wonders whether there is something like this here. Wait a minute, there's a little bit in my notes on Joseph's session: here it is, I did miss out a little. Joseph said of Jo: 'He eats more than me. I look after him quite well but we're not always the same, when I'm happy he's often sad.' Then Joseph gave that manic grin at me (you all know the one), and went on, 'now you can see I'm happy, but you can't see him, can you?'

J.A. That's marvellous, isn't it!

Myself: I replied, 'I only know what you tell me about Jo.'

J.A. Joseph is one of the children who will ask for more food, an extra helping, knowing in advance that he won't eat it. And it seems to me that this might be Jo's portion, or to make sure that Jo has enough.

It may well have been difficult to follow this discussion, but I feel that it is of value especially because of Joseph and Jo, and also since it gives some kind of picture of a treatment team reporting in this particular way.

The question now is, will Joseph have a regression, in which he would hand over the care of little Jo to us; or will he continue to be a caretaker-self. Is this as far as he can go? Ideally, we would want him to have a regression, so that Jo could grow up and become Joseph, one whole person. Joseph himself claimed recently that Jo is growing.

My last piece of material concerns Robert, in the Cotswold Community, at the age of fifteen.

Robert was referred to me within the Community because people were worried about him. He came quite willingly, shy, evasive, but friendly. He said, 'Well, what shall we talk about, now I'm here?' I said, 'I thought we might talk about you, Robert.' 'Oh,' he replied, 'there are two of those.' His tone was almost casual. I suggested in an equally calm and commonplace way that he should tell me a bit about *both of them*. He went on to explain that there was the Robert whom I could see and talk with, but also there was the other one—a little boy about eight years old, always getting into mischief. He described how difficult he found the task of controlling the little one. As far as he knew, there had always been the two of them —the little one was delinquent and got very excited: the big one was quiet, shy and withdrawn. Robert said: 'What worries me is that I'll soon be leaving here, and imagine the other one getting out at home or at work. There's nothing I can do for him—I've wondered about a youth club, but they don't *play*, not his way, just games and all that.' I could only sympathize: how could he have a regression at this point? How could he hand over the care of the little one—so much younger than eight years old—to us? Robert said, hesitatingly: 'I've had one idea. Do you think when I'm older and can get married, that my wife would look after him?' I said that this was a real possibility, that many marriages work on this sort of basis, but that it would be important to let the girl know about his little self before they were married. He agreed, and we talked round this.

On a later occasion, he told me, 'I've decided to get rid of him' (the little self), 'I'd get on better without him.' I begged him not to do this: I pointed out that he was talking about destroying his real self. He said, 'I can't keep him any longer.'

He did not want to see me again for some weeks. Then he asked to do so. This time he talked about leaving the Community, and described his mixed feelings. Just as he was going, he exclaimed, 'All the same, if I had a son of my own in trouble, I'd want him to come here.'

My object in putting together this patchwork has been to underline the terrifying fact that unless suitable treatment can be provided, a syndrome of deprivation is unlikely to alter. So a sixteen-year-old can continue to live exactly as he did at the age of two. One could make a similar patchwork from any of the syndromes of deprivation which I have listed. Such a child can be passed from person to person, from place to place, actually conscious of his needs but unable to communicate. This tragedy is not inevitable: we are being given the chance to do something about it.

7
Students with special needs,
1970

I read this to a child care group at Westcliff-on-Sea who brought to the subject a great deal of experience and thought. It seems to me important to realize and accept that many young people, although they may have considerable emotional problems, may with support have a lot to offer in the field of child care.

One could say with truth that every student has special needs, some of which we can meet, others which must be firmly handed back to the student; others, again, which do not surface, concerning which we may speculate, but about which we might not choose to communicate to the student for various good reasons. It is this last category which I am going to consider in this paper, because students with such needs are often precisely the borderline people about whom one asks oneself, 'Should they be coming into the field of child care?' 'Helping other people to help us', chapter 8 in *Therapy in Child Care,* was an attempt to describe the problems which inevitably turn up during supervision, and which really do stem from the students' own needs, rather than from other sources.

I am troubled by the split between experience and conceptualization, which tends to result from periods of practical work followed or preceded by study. Ideally, in this field, I would like to see experience followed by realization leading *at once* to communication and subsequent conceptualization–all taking place in the same place within the student's working day, within the context, in fact. The 'special needs' which I am thinking about would be more readily recognized, I believe, in these circumstances. Perhaps, however, we can approximate to such a way of working, within the framework of the student's supervision during placement–this is a diagnostic opportunity in terms of *need assessment*. Students are going to become staff: just as children need to be diagnosed on a basis of need, so do staff. There has to be an emotional economy in a place, and resources for provision must not be squandered.

As I see it, we have no right to expect students (or ourselves, for the matter of that) to have no special emotional needs, however minimal: but equally, we must be able to recognize and estimate emotional cost to others having to meet such needs – not only colleagues, but also children, however indirectly. This cost has got to be balanced realistically against the contribution such a person may be able to make to the life and work of the total group in a residential place. I am not saying that the more disturbed a student may be the greater will be the strain on the group potential for meeting needs. This is not necessarily so, since many very disturbed people may be highly organized and defended, so that, in a dreadful way they have no conscious needs and make no demands on others. (Indeed, often such apparently self-contained young people are envied by others, and their illness remains unrecognized until serious breakdown takes place.) There are many more obviously disturbed students who, one can see, will present many difficulties and whose needs must be met wherever they may be; who, all the same, have gifts and skills and whose insight may be of value. These are the borderline cases to which I have referred.

What should we as supervisors say to such people? How do we help them, advise them, and report on them to others? Very often these disturbed – but probably valuable – students are themselves emotionally deprived: something has gone wrong at the beginning of their lives, so that they have not had enough experience as babies to build adequate *selves*. In other words there will be gaps in their experience which have left gaps in their ego-functioning. The only treatment which can be of use to any such deprived person is provision of primary experience, either in the course of their lives through deep and dependent personal relationships, or through actual therapeutic treatment (very difficult to obtain). Now, I am not suggesting for a moment that we should provide such treatment for students, nor that we should hope that their needs can be met in this way as staff in child care units; although this may well be the student's own not so unconscious hope, and this hope may have a lot to do with motivation in his or her wish to work in the field of child care. It may, however, be worth while to consider the possibility of planning support for this kind of person, by conscious supplementation of functioning in those areas where the student's ego is missing or inadequate.

I remember one such student, working in a therapeutic school for several months: this was a very gifted and intelligent girl, well qualified and with considerable experience (on an advanced course in the United States). Jane was in most ways an ideal student, of whom we all had a high opinion and whom we respected. From time to time, however, perhaps once in two weeks, Jane would fail to get up in the morning, and would spend the day in bed: on the following morning she would reappear, with a graceful apology for her absence–but no explanation! You will know the irritation and resentment this sort of phenomenon can arouse –Jane's very lack of guilt and anxiety made matters worse. I was fairly certain that these days in bed were in fact 'mini-breakdowns' into regression, really needed by Jane and therefore not a matter of conflict for her. On the other hand, Jane was exploiting others in a split-off sort of way, which enabled her to avoid personal communication and personal responsibility for her survival technique. Obviously this was the tip of an iceberg, and something so well established that change of pattern was not likely to take place without tremendous emotional upheaval. Jane to some extent counted on collusive anxiety among her colleagues: the fear of losing her very real contribution could induce them to close their eyes to her 'departures'.

Following thought and consultation with the team of the therapeutic school, I decided to talk about this problem in its manifest form with Jane. The latent form would be dangerous for anyone of us to approach–it would open up the whole area of her early deprivation, of which we knew nothing. So I talked to Jane about the *reality* of her need to have these days in bed, making it clear to her that I completely accepted the subjective reality of this need. I said all this, sitting on her bed, on such a day. I felt as though I was going through a sound barrier, and expected a sonic boom: she certainly felt threatened and resentful, but my acceptance of the reality of her need gave her some assurance. By *manifest* content of non-functioning areas, I mean what one can see in objective reality: Jane really objectively stayed in bed. The *latent* content of this behaviour would be the *meaning* of staying in bed, for her, deeply rooted in her unconscious, and only to be reached in a treatment setting. Nothing would be more dang-

erous than interpretation of the need, even supposing the interpretation might be correct. A communicated recognition of the
need is a very different matter, and can even be eventually of therapeutic value.

I stressed to Jane that I recognized her need to go to bed on
certain days, but also that I felt this must be communicated to
others, to be considered as a practical problem requiring a solution. I said that eventually she might not need this withdrawal, but
that in the meantime this was something with which she and all
of us must live. She claimed that she had never talked about this
before, and that others had not challenged her right to withdraw.
I assured her that this right was not being challenged, but that
plans must be made, communication must be established so that
other people could and would—consciously and willingly—stand
in for her. In the end, such arrangements were made: the other
members of the team were much less resentful in response to
Jane's less defended position. Jane herself began consciously
to accept the split-off 'gap' as being in herself, in so far that she
could accept responsibility for her withdrawals and became able
to communicate such a state of non-functioning as soon as she
reached awareness of an impending breakdown. Although she
was unable to alter this pattern, she became much more conscious
of it, so that shortly before her placement came to an end, she
could discuss the possibility of telling future employing agencies
about the problem—as she would do, after all, if she suffered from
severe attacks of asthma. Many people, of course, achieve the same
results as Jane, quite unconsciously, through some psychosomatic
symptom, which is unlikely to be challenged by others as an escape
route.

I do not feel that such steps should be taken by us unless we
are confident that the student can offer so much to the place that
he or she is *worth* this considerable trouble. We must, however,
bear in mind the fact that many apparently down-to-earth sensible
students have made a 'flight to reality', and are consequently
quite out of touch with their own inner reality and unable to gain
real insight; they are unable to achieve empathy with children
or grown-ups.

Other deprived students may appear to function successfully,
but are in fact delinquent. Delinquency is not so easy to recognize

when there is no obvious stealing or other dishonest behaviour. Delinquent personalities can hide behind competence and charm: gradually one starts to feel uneasy. Children are seduced by such a person; grown-ups are manipulated. There is often a paranoid attitude, linked with pairing: this sort of pairing is really merger.[1] The delinquent student merges with a suitable unintegrated child –a host, as it were–and takes up an isolated position with the child *against* the rest of the grown-ups, children in the group. It is my view that no such student should remain in the field of child care. There is nothing to gain by trying to help this kind of person in a unit. I would ask for his or her removal, giving my reasons. It is most unlikely that a delinquent grown-up will evolve, because there are too many secondary gains from delinquency. Some agency must deal with his problem, but *not* the staff of a unit caring for deprived children–*we* cannot meet his needs.

Another deprivation syndrome which I have met among students is the kind of intellectually brilliant person who has had to use his intellect as a defence against his emotional life. Such a person is usually omnipotent and narcissistic, sure of his ability to solve any problem by intellectual means, and consequently scornful of intuition and insight (I am inclined to think of insight as informed intuition). This kind of student is a constant source of irritation to all: his sheer intellectual ability can be a threat, and his ability to argue himself out of untenable positions by the use of rather dotty logic can be actually destructive. This student certainly has special needs, of which he is usually unaware because of massive defences. The supervision of such a student can be utterly exhausting and frustrating, unless one takes measures from the first to control the situation. I personally, as soon as I recognize an extreme intellectual defence, insist from the first on basing all discussion on the student's actual experiences in the place. Here again, I do not interpret, except once removed, as it were: in the material which emerges the student will probably be able to stand some gain of insight. This kind of person may be deeply concerned for the children in the place, and even relatively free emotionally in regard to them, but the intellectual defence will be mobilized

---

[1] I use the word 'merger' to describe a symbiotic bond, where one person merges with another, or a group, in order to escape responsibility of identity.

against parental figures or in sibling rivalry. Providing that insight can be gained gradually, and the supervisor is not trapped into a punitive attitude, such a student can continue to evolve into a successful worker.

So far I have been talking for the most part about endemic pathological states in students. There can be special needs which are occasional emergencies and which need to be met at once: for example, shock. It is not unusual for a student, especially in a unit catering for disturbed children or adolescents, to be sailing along quite successfully as far as we can see, only to break down in one way or another at the end of a few weeks. Usually warm concern and support are all that is needed, with opportunities for communication. I have found it useful to warn students of this possibility of stress. Sometimes such a breakdown is not only shock, but an uncovering of deep disturbance, triggered off by reflection in the children. There can, however, be pockets of disturbance in people which are usually fairly well insulated, and the same approach as for shock can re-establish the necessary defences. On the whole, I do not, as a supervisor, encourage students to talk about their own personal lives, but there should be a time and a place for this when they need urgently to communicate something to us about themselves, often on a basis of trust in our reliability in regard to the children. Therapeutic listening with a minimum of comment can be a kind of first aid at these moments.

If one finds that a student is quite unable to cope emotionally in some specific area–for example, the management of panic in children–I would suggest that, rather as with non-functioning areas, we accept the reality of this specific inability, communicate our acceptance to the student, and see to it that he is not expected to manage such situations except in a secondary role.

You will realize that I am thinking here about students who are not fully integrated as individuals. These are the ones with the really special needs: they can be valuable workers eventually, but in the meantime they can only too easily collect the roles of proteges or scapegoats. I have met them in every area of caring for children. Their gifts arouse envy and their underfunctioning arouses resentment, but some of them can do valuable work; and in all of them is the potential to evolve.

8
Need assessment – I
Finding a basis, 1970

The Home Office asked me to run a workshop on need assessment—from dawn till dusk!—at Bournemouth, as part of a course for experienced workers. This was an immensely stimulating and exciting experience, and we were all exhausted by the end of it! There have been several workshops on need assessment since this first one, including an occasion when Barbara Chumbley and I worked together with a course over two days.

The notes which follow are written from a highly personal point of view, and from a position outside the field of child care. I could have attempted to make some sort of survey of means of assessment that are in use here and in other countries. I could have advocated this method and deprecated that; wished for this or that sociometric scale; or groaned over some projection technique: what I have actually done is to make basic assumptions to assume that any human being making an assessment of the state of any other human being is faced inevitably by the same difficulties within himself, whatever techniques are employed in the task of assessment. Just at the moment, so much is in a state of flux: presently, no doubt our work will reset into various stereotyped forms. But here and now, there is an element of choice, just because there is also an element of uncertainty. We are thinking today especially about the problems attending assessment at the point of taking into care. Perhaps the 'winds of change' are even altering the meaning of 'care'.

The word 'assessment' has a final ring; there is something absolute about the statement or series of statements which may alter the entire life of an individual human being. Those people who make assessments are in an omnipotent position: how they move and countermove will depend on many factors—and ultimately the arrangements of their words written on paper will tend to lead to instant action, since in the circumstances, if such action were not needed there would not be in the first place a request for an assessment. In other words, the process of assessment is usually required to deal with crisis. The action necessary (whatever this may be) results from a state of emergency in the life of a person within a group. You will have noticed that, so far, I have not used the word 'child'. I think I am especially anxious that we should be thinking of a *person* who is a child; who was a baby and who will become a grown-up, but who throughout all his life should be respected as a person. In this connection, I was considering the word 'pity' recently and wondered why I dislike the sound of 'pity': I concluded that 'pity' is not a feeling which of necessity involves 'respect'. I found myself preferring 'compassion', which–for me, anyhow–implies respect for the human being who evokes my compassion. 'Pity' has overtones of patronage–it comes from above, downwards. You will realize that I am wondering about the attitudes which various workers must bring to the task of assessment. I am remembering a report made by an army psychiatrist on a seven-year-old boy who had caused a lot of trouble: in this report the psychiatrist described the child as 'a potential psychopath' and I am asking myself whether he really thought about the possible effect of such a dangerous and final assessment on the rest of the boy's life.

A fifteen-year-old was sent to an approved school from a classifying school. He was described as a case of school truancy. I read the various reports and recommendations, dating from when he was seven years old. His elder brother had been murdered in Orchard Street–this was stated in one report. In another report his truancy was described: this had started when he was seven, and the school from which he played truant was the 'Orchard Street School'. *No connection* in all the intervening years had been made by the reporting agencies between the street in which his brother was murdered, and the school *in the same street* from which he fled. Nevertheless, all the information was there, clearly to be read in the two separate reports, linking the murder with what was, of course, an unrecognized school phobia. Here at least were clues which could eventually be found which helped us to assess the boy's final state. Often, however, there are no real facts available, either because those people from whom we are trying to collect information are inadequate or because they really do not know what happened during the critical years of the child's early child-hood. A boy of about eight who was coming to see me from time to time, wondered about the curious pock marks which covered his face. Eventually he and I realized that these must have been self-inflicted, in the course of terrible deprivation in early child-hood. It was not until much later that we found confirmation (through a chance meeting with a nurse): for months, as a toddler, he had torn at his own face with his fingernails. The pock marks were there for all to see, but there was no mention of this evidence of despair in any of the detailed reports. Parents, teachers and others are often themselves in the whirlpool of the crisis, full of guilt and anxiety, which made their reporting highly subjective.

I remember how, long ago, a little boy was referred to the Mulberry Bush by a child guidance clinic. He was described by his mother as violent and dangerous: she gave detailed descriptions of his disturbed behaviour and eventually he was sent to us, having formally been ascertained maladjusted. Actually it was soon clear that he was indeed a very disturbed child, although we were puzzled by the fact that he did not present the behaviour pattern drawn in such detail by his mother. At a later stage when I took this up with her one day, she suddenly revealed to me that she had been describing her husband's behaviour at home: it seemed to her that only by attaching this to her little son could she report her husband's maladjustment without disloyalty to him!

With the decrease in the number of court orders, the positions and attitudes of parents of delinquent children may be radically altered. We can hope that parents will become less guilty and anxious, and consequently less defended, so that they may be free to consider their own and their children's problems more objectively with us, provided that we can give them adequate support.

In order to make any kind of assessment in regard to a person, information must be collected by other people from other people and then communicated by people to people. This final communication is bound to be influenced by all the current factors operating in the lives of the many people involved—above all, by the sense of urgency, because of the 'crisis' climate of which I have already spoken. All the *feelings* of the worried people engulfed in the crisis, are going to be in the assessment and also all the feelings of the workers who are making the assessment

There is a famous French film about this problem, concerning the jury in a murder trial—a study of the effects of their current problems on their judgment. The parents (if there are parents) will be trying to deal with guilt and inadequacy. The workers may be feeling a different sort of guilt, if they are in fact having to take a child away from his home and family—however inadequate these may be.

There will be the feelings evoked by the child's personality in those who are dealing with him at such a moment, and also *his* reaction to the strangers who have come into his life which will affect his behaviour. Given such an emotional climate, it may be difficult to sort out the objective reality. The history presented by the parents may omit much, and distort even more (for example, the mother of battered babies). The child may present a false picture of himself, because he will be under great stress: even his intelligence may be blurred by underfunctioning due to emotional disturbance. A disturbed boy of high average intelligence was involved in a delinquent act which brought him before a magistrate's court. He was retested at this point (at the request of the magistrate) and his intelligence now appeared to be well below average at 80. A year later, by which time he had started to respond to treatment, his good intelligence was, on further testing, once again in evidence.

Of course, in a reception centre much of this confusion can be to some extent sorted out; but even here the child may not be able to communicate his needs and his real personality, either by what he says or what he does.

I think we are accepting too easily a process of a structured kind, which gives everyone concerned the illusion of solving problems and making appropriate recommendations, when actually we may not have reached the real problems; and our recommendations—however appropriate—may be impossible to implement. I am in favour of communicating and tolerating doubt: it is rare in assessments—of disturbed children, for example—to meet words like 'possibly', 'perhaps', 'we think', or even 'we do not understand'.

Most of my experience of assessments has been of those made by child guidance clinic teams and these are usually excellent valid reports, but even such highly professional teams—who may not be working in a crisis climate—can make mistakes. For example: a frozen delinquent boy was referred to us as 'deeply depressed'. Within a few months there was dramatic evidence that the so-called depression was only a state of hibernation between one delinquent explosion and the 'next, which suddenly took place for all to see. His delinquent exploits had up till this point escaped discovery. I believe that such mistakes are inevitable; that no reporting can be entirely objective, and that the information collected in a situation of stress may well be invalid; but I am not supposing for a moment that we can *avoid* error, that we can ever be sure that we are making a correct assessment of a breakdown in a constellation of lives. I am only urging that we should support each other in the toleration of doubt, and recognize the inadequacy of the knowledge on which we must depend in order to take action which will affect the future life of the person concerned to an extent which we are in no position to calculate.

What will be the population of a community home? How are we going to judge whether such placement will meet the needs of *this* child at *this* time? What can such a home offer? Are we able to classify children in such a way that, in taking them into care for the first time we can ensure that they will be obtaining *appropriate* care? Some of you may have seen the devastating Robertson film called '*John*,'[1] in which a normal integrated toddler is placed by his father in a residential nursery, in a group of institutionalized little children who are cared for by young nursery nurses working on a shift system. By the end of seventeen days John is destroyed by his environment, perhaps never to recover. The caring was in itself kind, but ill-planned and inadequate; nevertheless the same standard of care in a group of integrated toddlers would not have been so disastrous (this placement was, of course, planned by the parents). Are we going to be able to *plan* emotional environments or shall we in the event, like John's father, have to use whatever place we can find?

I feel we should be able to decide whether we are going to mix integrated and unintegrated children in one living group, or whether we may plan in such a way as to have integrated groups

[1] See footnote p. 72.

and unintegrated groups, with two distinct kinds of provision based on need. I realize that decisions will rest with the social workers and the children's department: even a case which comes before the magistrates will return to the children's officer. Up till now, the decision as to whether a delinquent boy would go to an approved school or a school for the maladjusted often depended on the particular views of a probation officer. Who will now decide his placement, and on what basis? What specialized knowledge will immediately be available to a children's department? Will there be enough consultation available with the responsible key people in the child's life—the teacher, the general practitioner, the health visitor? How much time will be available to consider the doubtful cases—whether or no to take a little child into care? Often there will not be much room for doubt, but it must sometimes be difficult to decide: who, exactly, will reach this decision? Suppose that an unintegrated aggressive boy goes into a reception home, unable to make relationships: will he meet there normal children awaiting appropriate placement? What will be the effect on the normal, integrated children, who will be distressed and vulnerable in any case because of a strange environment?

You will understand that I know very little about the actual process of taking a child into care: there may be immediate answers to my questions. But perhaps questions which have been answered in one context may be asked again in another, even though the original answers may still turn out to be valid. Certainly, in the field of residential placement of maladjusted children, I have the feeling that placement in a school is too often the discovery of a vacant place, rather than the meeting of the needs of the particular child and the matching of child to school. This is not a criticism of assessment, there is an inevitable collusion of which we are all to some extent guilty, in which we *accept* that something actually essential is not available, and assess accordingly; for example, —the fact that there are not enough adolescent units. I would hope that we are free to insist that assessment and recommendation should have in mind *what is needed* over and above *what is available*.

Perhaps the community homes will be able to provide a considerable variety of provision around a campus: a flexible range which will enable a child to move from one unit to another on basis of need fulfilment. For example: an 'intensive care' unit in terms of emotional provision might be able to give treatment (primary provision) to a child for a comparatively short period, followed by skilled but less intensive care in a more normal environment.

Since need assessments were first introduced in the Mulberry Bush and the Cotswold Community we have taken a further step and are now evolving a referral need assessment made by the referring agency (a classifying school, reception centre, or whatever) in communication with the placement under conisderation.

It would seem that we can never assess need sufficiently early, and rarely under normal conditions. I believe that assessment centres should be run on the lines of day hospitals, with children living in their own homes whenever possible during assessment; we would be much more likely to make accurate assessments in such circumstances. There will, of course, be a considerable difference between a referral need assessment and an ongoing need assessment (which will be one of a series). In both cases all need assessments must, in my view, be made by a group, *never* by an individual collecting information or depending upon interview procedure.

There is a useful word which I have only met as a traffic term, used on main roads: this is the word 'clearway'. I feel that we need a clearway for discussion, without the pressure of crisis, which can so easily force us to reach decisions in assessment which may not be appropriate for this person who is about to become 'a child in care'.

9
Need assessment – II
Making an assessment, 1970

The particular kind of need assessment which I shall be discussing
came into being as the result of a collection of experiences, working
in a consultant role in a school for deeply disturbed and deprived
children (the Mulberry Bush) and in a therapeutic community
which has evolved from an approved school (the Cotswold Community). At the Mulberry Bush I evolved a type of reporting which
I called 'context profiles'.[1] When making a context profile, the
whole team consider one child, chosen by the team, for a week.
Each member describes any actual personal experiences which he
has had with this child: observations are not allowed. I myself
have a therapeutic session with the child concerned during the
week. All notes are brought to the school secretary, who then
types the material and circulates the notes to the team and to me,
so that we can meet at the end of the week to discuss our experiences, drawing conclusions from the material and gearing a
treatment programme to the needs which become apparent.
Donald Winnicott made the valuable comment that, by using this
method, the team can for an instant see the *whole* child, because all
the 'bits' are brought together in the profile–not only the bits of
the child, but also all our feelings about him. Following the dis-

[1] See *Therapy in Child Care*, ch. 10

cussion, all the notes are arranged in a classification on context: thus all 'getting up' experiences are together and 'mealtimes' and 'bedtimes' are treated in the same way. Since each person may have very different experiences, the outcome is a study in depth of the child and ourselves, attempting to avoid the snares of pseudo-objectivity[1].

From the work on one child, light is often thrown on the needs and treatment of others. The context profile discussion is recorded on tape (the notes are typed in advance) and the whole profile is arranged as described, by our secretary, Mrs Connie Barrett. Ultimately we have something valuable both to us, to psychiatrists, and to newcomers to the team. The work, however, is time-consuming and nowadays we decide to do a profile only when we are especially puzzled and concerned about a particular child. I found that in order to make use of a context profile (at a clinic, for example), I needed to make an analysis. This I did by asking myself certain questions, to which I found answers in the material. Working in parallel at the Cotswold Community, I showed the teams of the various houses how to make context profiles. Here there are four teams (instead of one, as at the Mulberry Bush) and very little secretarial help. There is, inevitably, more coming and going of the adolescent delinquents (because of court orders, up to the present) and in any case, I only meet these groups at the Cotswold once weekly, whereas I meet the Bush team twice weekly. All these factors made the task of writing profiles very difficult.

At the Bush selection has always been based on primary deprivation, so that we are carefully selecting unintegrated children for treatment. At the Cotswold referrals are mixed—integrated and unintegrated—with a much larger unintegrated group than we originally realized. We have found that it is essential to classify boys on arrival as integrated or unintegrated as soon as possible, and it was in order to make this possible that I tried to plan a need assessment. I hoped this would categorize, consider the stage of integration reached, and formulate needs and the treatment to meet these needs.

I decided to use exactly the questions which I ask myself when

[1]See chapter 5.

analysing a profile. This meant employing a certain amount of terminology, but I improvised a glossary (I find terms necessary as a kind of shorthand; otherwise one is employing essays instead of terms). I reached the decision to use these particular questions because I had arrived at them through actual relevant experience: in the event, they proved of use. No doubt in time, we may ask some more questions and omit existing ones: the whole idea is still at a workshop stage, but perhaps for that reason it calls for discussion and experiment. We may also find clearer terms, but since these words are the ones which I employ at present, I have let them stand, with explanations.

CLASSIFICATION

The process of arriving at a need assessment is described in detail below. I have tried to approach the problem of meeting the child's needs–whatever these may be–by classification (rather than by considering his symptoms). I think it will always be necessary for a senior worker to lead such a group discussion, asking and explaining the questions, and recording the answers. There can be no 'yes' or 'no' answers: all replies must be based on actual experiences with the child. We have found that this kind of assessment helps us in planning for the child's management and care.

A need assessment in no way replaces other assessments (case history, intellectual ability and so on), but I find it a valuable addition to other information.

The questions in this assessment can only be answered for the first time by a group of people who are living with the child, and have been doing so for at least three or four weeks: they must understand that this is a *first* need assessment–others will be necessary in order to meet the child's evolving needs. Only a group of resident workers can draw on the kind of experience essential to this type of assessment.

The questions may seem odd at first, but they seem to obtain the kind of information necessary, and workers quickly become accustomed to this approach. A need assessment usually takes an hour of group work to complete.

NEED ASSESSMENT

Classification

Is this child integrated as a person, or is he unintegrated? To judge this, one should ask oneself:

(*a*) *Does he panic?* By panic, I mean a state of unthinkable anxiety —almost a physical condition. (Many so-called 'temper tantrums' are panics.)

(*b*) *Does he disrupt?* By this, I mean does he disrupt a group activity or a happening between two other people?

It would appear, from evidence so far, that the presence of panic and disruption fairly frequently in a child's life justifies us in considering him, for the present, as being unintegrated.

If you are sure that panic and disruption are rarely experienced, then go on to the next section, in which the needs of integrated children are considered.

UNINTEGRATED CHILDREN

If he seems to be unintegrated, go on to the next question.

1. *What is the syndrome of deprivation?* This can be judged by answers to the following questions. What is the state of feelings in this child in regard to

(*a*) personal guilt

This refers to concern; to what one could call healthy guilt—not a fear of being punished or found out, but an acceptance of a personal responsibility for harm done to others, of a kind which can lead to making reparation.

(*b*) Dependence on people or a person

(*c*) Merger

This is the way in which some children become merged with one other or with a group (a typically delinquent phenomenon).

(*d*) Empathy

I like to think of this as being a capacity to imagine what it must feel like to be in someone else's shoes, while remaining in one's own.

(*e*) Stress

How does this child appear to deal with feelings of stress?

(*f*) Communication
Does he *really* communicate, or does he just chatter in a sterotyped way?

(*g*) Identification
Does he, for example, seem to model himself on a grown-up he admires, or on another child? Be careful not to confuse this with *merger*.

(*h*) Depression
Is he sometimes very depressed, or is he indifferent, or always apparently cheerful? Is he at times deeply sad? There is a kind of state of low level of consciousness—just 'ticking over'—sometimes even in deprived children, which I call 'hibernation' and which should not be confused with depression.

(*i*) Aggression
—verbal and physical.

2. *What is his capacity for play?*
(*a*) Narcissistic
Does he play a lot alone, with pleasure?
(*b*) Transitional
Does he, for example, make use of a transitional object?
(*c*) Pre-oedipal
Does he usually like to play with one other, usually a grown up?
(*d*) Oedipal
Does he play with more than one grown up at a time?
(*e*) Post-oedipal
Does he play with other children, able to keep rules, and so on?
(See *Therapy in Child Care*, ch. 11.

3. *What is his capacity for learning*—in every sort of learning situation? Does he learn from experience?

4. *What is his capacity for self preservation?* Is he accident prone? Does he take care of himself and his belongings? Does he seem to value himself?

From the material it is usually quite possible to make a good guess at the *stage of integration* reached. The stages are as follows (see *Therapy in Child Care,* pp. 99–101):

(*a*) Frozen
(*b*) Archipelago
(*c*) False-self
(*d*) Caretaker-self

(On this 'inside diagnosis' a need assessment can be made. There is nothing *absolute* about such recommendations; we cannot be certain, but this assessment gives us a foundation for a treatment programme.) In general, one could say that the needs of these categories are as follows:

(*a*) *Frozen.* Containment, especially of self-destructive areas. Mergers to be interrupted.
Delinquent action to be anticipated – essentially, *confrontation in advance,* i.e. knowing what the child is going to do.
Acting out to be converted into communication.
Dependence on grown-ups to be established.
Delinquent excitement to be changed into oral greed.
Depression to be reached, and supported, following a capacity for personal guilt.
Open communication – with one; with others.

(*b*) *Archipelago.* To relate one ego-functioning islet to others, through communication.
Containment of non-functioning areas, e.g. panics.
Support and encouragement of any functioning areas.
Provision of localized regression where needed, with reliable adaptation.

(*c*) *False-self.* Containment of chaos within the shell. Provision of regression, always planned and localized, with reliable adaptation. Symbolic communication.

(*d*) *Caretaker-self.* Provision for localized regression, reached through cooperation with the 'caretaker', in the care of the real self.
Symbolic communication.
Localized adaptations with as much communication as possible between grown-ups and child.
Functioning areas should be strongly backed.

The particular form which such primary provision should take will depend on the personality of the child and on what he indicates, however indirectly. There will need to be *verbal* and *pre-verbal* communication.

There must be reassessment quite frequently—whenever fundamental evolvement is noted, or indeed any real change for better or worse.

Integrated children

Where the original classification indicates that the child is integrated, the position is very different and need assessment is more complex. We can say with certainty, however, that an integrated, neurotic child will need from us:

Ego support, especially where there is under-functioning: e.g. with doubtful, anxious children.

Reliable parental figures, on to whom he can transfer the unresolved conflicts in regard to his parents.

Ways in which he can make positive use of aggression.

'Open' communication, and the opportunities for conversion of acting-out into verbal communication.

Encouragement and opportunity to accept responsibility as an individual in a group (here 'shared responsibility' becomes very important).

Acceptance of reparation, and help to reach this reparation.

Help in modifying a harsh super-ego.

Nevertheless, need assessment for integrated children will be far more individual and must be considered in great detail.

Notes

1. I have considered especially the needs of unintegrated children, because so many of the children we are trying to help are in fact only partially integrated, and these are the ones who present the greatest problems of management.
2. Please bear in mind that this is only an experimental draft which will need to be developed as a result of experience. Suggestions and alterations will be needed.
3. I have said nothing about symptoms, because this fails to reach *needs*. Children come to us because of their needs, not their symptoms.

Here is a need assessment on Lilian, carried out by the Bush team working with me. (At the Cotswold Community, some teams are doing need assessments by themselves, so that we can discuss the material when we meet.)

Classification

Presence of panic and disruption: Both present, therefore *unintegrated*.

1. What is the state of feelings in Lilian in regard to
   (a) *Guilt* (guilt really means concern). There is a capacity for feelings of personal guilt which shows in compunction in regard to wrong or hurtful things which she has done, which does not *seem* to stem from fear of punishment.
   (b) *Dependence* on person or people (this category includes trust). Lilian is able to be dependent on individuals and also is able to be dependent on the Mulberry Bush. (Example: it is not now necessary for her to be sick on returning to the school; she does not have to test all the time, because expectations are established.)
   (c) *Merger*. Yes, she does merge. More with individuals, but ocassionally with the group. One could use the term 'passive merger'—she passively accepts being used.
   (d) *Empathy*. There is a possible capacity for empathy. Sometimes, perhaps, it might be projective identification.
   (e) *Stress*. Under stress, Lilian is liable to break down into states of panic rage, although this is rather less in evidence than at an earlier stage. (When in one of these states she will bite, she will spit—it will be all over her face, she will throw around everything in the room.) She can sometimes contain and communicate stress.
   (f) *Communication*. Lilian is capable of direct communication: at certain stages it is possible for her to communicate even when under stress.
   (Example of direct communication: when the group came back from a school outing, when the children were very tired, Lilian said, 'The trouble is, I hate my sister and she hates me.')

Query as to whether her long monologues are communication or a defence against communication. There is considerable confusion–sometimes there are flights of associations based on the immediate context or environment. Sometimes mode of communication resembles that of one very old.

(g) *Identification.* Her mannerisms, the way she walks, seem very like those of an elderly person. Lilian does not much appear to be identified with people here; identifications (what there are) come from her past and her background, rather than from anything that has happened here.

(h) *Depression.* Very sad a lot of the time: tinged with self-pity. She rather enjoys sorrowful, tearful, woeful things; enjoys the feeling of being sad. (When the saddest things are on television her face is lit up with pleasure!) This is more likely to be primary masochism.

(i) *Aggression.* Her form of movement could be seen as fairly aggressive. Not really aggressive unless provoked–aggression seen in self defence. (Example: Sheila slapped Lilian's face and Lilian called Sheila a 'black bitch', Sheila slapped her face then for this, Lilian again called Sheila a black bitch, and this just went on and on.) Lilian displays a certain courage to the point of living dangerously, but seems quite unaware of her place in the hierarchy of children. The words 'angry' and 'outraged' apply to her attitudes.

2. What is her capacity for play?
   Narcissistic; mainly narcissistic, just beginning to be able to play on her own but in a group–but this is still alone.

3. What is her capacity for learning?
   She does not seem very able to learn from experience; she cannot avoid disaster even when shown step by step what is going to happen to her; she goes on with her basic assumptions. There is some learning capacity in group: she can do simple sums and write figures, although she is unable to read or write. Although there is some learning capacity for number work, in general she has a very low capacity in all areas. Must take into consideration her low I.Q. and deafness–both of these factors could aggravate this inability to learn. (With very high

motivation, some learning has taken place—she can now decide what she wishes to spend her 5p on in the tuck shop.)

4. What is her capacity for self preservation?
Lilian shows signs of physical self preservation, but not of emotional self preservation. She does use adults to protect her, is not accident prone.

Stage of integration reached:

False-self. This after much discussion but within the confines of the headings; given, the collected data indicated false-self child, but with some evidence of a real core.

Need assessment recommendation:

We should support any area that is functioning. Containment of chaos within the shell. Provision of regression, always planned and localized, with reliable adaptations. Symbolic communication.

Other recommendations:

This child's I.Q. is so low that this could be the wrong school for her; there is the added problem of her deafness. One cannot overlook, however, that whatever her problems here, they will be equally valid in, say, an E.S.N. school.

The strain, for Lilian, of being here with children of higher intelligence, could be too great and her need could be somewhere where the whole thing would be geared to a lower I.Q. and to her deafness.

Despite the handicaps she has clearly benefited from being here, and it might not be in her best interests to lose what she obviously gains from the Mulberry Bush School and us.

How much regression has Lilian had here, and has she indicated a need for regression? We assume that for a false-self child to recover, there must be regression—they have got to go to bits and then come together and start off again. From the fact that she tries to get in on the act (i.e. wanting to have German measles when Susan had them: saying she had wet the bed, etc.) it could well be that she is looking for some means of regression.

Is Lilian able to indicate adaptations, and are there any available for her? Felt she would like a good adaptation made available: there is quite a bit of regression going on around and she takes full advantage of this.

The position is that is she is going to need a real regression, a lot of adaptation and a lot of very early experience, very definite focused primary provision for quite a time; this would be the only way in which this particular syndrome would evolve: equally, we may feel that this isn't something that we here can provide because of the added factors of the low I.Q. and the deafness, which may make it really impossible, if so, then we will have to think of other placement. If, however, she is to stay here, it could only be on a basis of real regression, and to what extent this is possible, and how, with someone like this, I don't know. One would say the need assessment is adaptation leading to regression with the beginning of integration following: a very big regression and then reforming, not reaching conceptualization (so many children do, after regression)–she would *realize* what she had been through, but she wouldn't be able to *think* it out. But she could make use of a regression.

You may be interested to know that, after the assessment, the team was in a better position to understand and meet Lilian's needs, and progress has been made in her treatment, so that it seems likely that she will stay with us, and that her regression will be reached.

You will notice that the first classification–whether integrated or unintegrated–is made on the presence or absence of panic and disruption. There is a further clue in the question relating to ego functioning, 'Is there a capacity for empathy?' (not to be confused with projective identification). Should one at that point find clear evidence of empathy, one should return to the question of panic and disruption, since it may be, for example, that acute but contained states of anxiety have been mistaken for panic.

You will also have noticed that we are primarily concerned with state of mind rather than behaviour. Symptoms turn up in discussion, but these–especially acting out–are considered as broken-down communications of state of mind; our treatment plans being based on the needs which the broken-down communications indicate.

Of course, in using need assessment within a residential unit, we assume that other appropriate information is already either in our possession, or at least readily available. A series of need assessments *can* only be used in a residential place by a team working together and living with the child. I suspect, from my own experience as a consultant, that a wealth of valuable material is available in any children's home, but that child care workers need a professional structure and discipline in order to communicate and organize reports which will lead to appropriate treatment programmes. This is equally true both in approved schools and in schools for maladjusted children.

Here is another need assessment, on a recovering boy, who was so unintegrated and dangerous on referral that we wondered whether we could hold him. He was on referral what I have termed an 'archipelago' child, who progressed to become a 'caretaker self', and is now precariously integrated. It is very interesting to see phases of development belonging to the first year of life, turning up during treatment.

BRUCE'S NEED ASSESSMENT

Integrated: Perhaps barely. Does not panic (psychotic area could be quite large). Disrupts in a very conscious way.

1. *Ego functioning*
   Feelings of
   (a) *Guilt.* Yes.
   (b) *Dependence.* Yes.
   (c) *Merger.* Very much diminishing—certainly meeting him, one gets a very clear impression of identity.
   (d) *Empathy.* Yes.
   (e) *Stress.* Depends very much on the relationship formed with grown-up with him at particular time. If he meets a stressful situation involving other children, he will now preserve himself: with a grown-up he can on occasions tend to trust in the grown-up to cope with the situation for him.

   More and more, when he is anxious, frightened or angry, this results in an inturned situation where he goes silent (what one could call an 'inplosion') and takes the trouble in with him, then, with encouragement, it comes out with a rush, shouting, i.e. an explosion. (He is further ahead than we could have ever hoped, when we think of all the ghastly things he used to do at the slightest stress.)

(*f*) *Communication*. Pretty good, both verbal and non-verbal: particularly non-verbal. He uses looks as a very conscious tool, gesture–he knows he has an expressive face, and uses it.

(*g*) *Identification*. Yes, in a positive sense. (With his group teacher and with his father, but as two clear and distinct things; he consciously separates group teacher (Brian) and father.)

(*h*) *Depression*. Yes–quite sad. Suggestion that manic flight could come in here, when he throws things, etc., much laughing, all a flight from feeling personal guilt and depression.

(*i*) *Aggression*. Yes. Incident with Bill and a very angry Bruce chasing him with a piece of glass: Robin felt on this occasion that Bruce would have used it if there had not been intervention. Still doubt really as to what Bruce may or may not do–and to what extent intervention on all occasions is justified. (This is a child who has been given cause for murderous rage at home; what this step-mother has made his father into is one of many reasons.) He is still capable of what seems to be less than conscious destruction.

(Comment from myself: A psychotic area of a person is something that is not capable of evolvement. The violent bit of him even might eventually be accepted by him and others as a mad bit, rather than an unintegrated bit.)

He tolerates his step-mother now, for the pleasure of being with his father.

2. What is his capacity for play?
Narcissistic. No longer: does not now play on his own with his soldiers, no longer plays with lots of little pieces but prefers one larger thing–a bike, a gun or a football.
Post-oedipal. Not over good, but he does manage.

3. What is his capacity for learning?
Academic. Had his step-mother not destroyed his pleasure in learning, he would be much more receptive. He could do

with time entirely alone with a teacher, when he is capable of learning a great deal very quickly. One needs to overcome his unpleasant associations with learning, and combine this with skilful teaching and he should flourish.

Reading: reading age has gone up $1\frac{1}{2}$ years in this last year, and 2 years in the previous year.

Numbers: he likes number work and is prepared to do it. He uses it as a medium of identification with his father (who is in electronics). He still has a relatively short attention span, which is a handicap.

Learning from experience. He is wily, aware, and knowledgeable, very quick. An example was concerned with the sheepdog trials at the church fete. Brian set out to explain the routine to Bruce as he might to his own son, who is aged six. Bruce interrupted, saying, 'Don't go on, it's a code.' He can pick up the whole notion or idea immediately–a great capacity for learning.

He provokes other children: he calls it 'starting trouble' I suggested that this is the only way he can get attention from his father at home, by 'starting trouble'. Father appears a very detached man. Feeling is that Bruce can now relate to a man, father is getting a transference as it were; evidence of more warmth from father on recent visit here. So able to communicate with father, and father is able to respond: emotional change in Bruce (rather than maturation) has made this possible. (I recalled the first meeting with Bruce and his father: it was chilling. There was no connection whatever between these two: this great tall man and this tiny little shrivelled up tadpole sitting at some distance from his father; and one couldn't see what on earth they had in connection with each other . . . although his father was concerned, worried about him, wanting to do something.)

4. What is his capacity for self preservation?
Very much more self preservative than he was. This seems to stem from when he deliberately cut himself deeply with a sharp balsa knife. Group teacher would have like to have made it a significant thing but was wary of doing so. When Bruce starts trouble now, it is consistently pointed out that he does more harm to himself than to other people; recently he has been able to say 'Why?' and we are able to go through the things that he

is doing to himself when he started these situations: now he is able to give up with a smile, grin or wink as a communication that he has not finally, irrevocably hurt himself that time. (I wondered if a lot of the going-on was to gain attention.... At one time he may have felt that the only way he could obtain attention from his father, or any man, was to hurt himself; hence his quite terrible accident-proneness when he first came to us. We really felt it was too dangerous for him, for us to keep him here.)

Capacity for self-preservation is now quite good, although there are moments when he contemplates suicide quite consciously: before it was not conscious but was as if something overwhelmed him; so there are still suicidal elements which could come into the mad bit of him. The suicide bit now tends to come when he is depressed or sad: he is fascinated by death. He is attempting to preserve himself, but the battle to maintain himself is great.

There is a refusal to grow, a refusal to get better.

SUMMARY

From the above material this would seem to be a more or less integrated child, with a mad area, who could be left permanently with a suicidal tendency, or a tendency to murder (this would be incredibly impulsive). These are dangers of which he must gradually, as he grows older and stronger, become more aware and be something of which he is conscious and can take precautions against.

The acquisition of knowledge is very important to him and with this he will achieve a great deal in his own eyes: a great boost to his morale. He has an incredible agility of mind.

Felt that if he could win an intellectual argument with his mother, this would make the world of difference to his self-esteem in the home situation: or, if he could teach his mother something (say, chess) and she could stand being taught by him—if this could be 'sold' to her as the most beneficial thing she could do, to allow him to teach her something . . . John doubted that she wanted to do anything beneficial. He has got to be put in a position where he is independent of her from this sort of standpoint, and able to hold his own.

I went through the listed needs of integrated children. Extra comment on 'Help in modifying a harsh super-ego', i.e. help in replacing the punitive super-ego, which he has certainly got, by a more benign one, which one hopes he will incorporate from his experiences with us.

Group teacher commented on his responsibility within group which is showing signs of developing. He was asked by another child in the group what the difference between a Big and a Small was. Bruce's reply was 'a small somebody starts something, and a big somebody stops it'.

About reparation, as this could be important: he will give a grudging 'sorry' with no heart in it whatsoever; there is no evidence that he feels concern.

One of the main things then is to help him to obtain, contain and make use of, as much knowledge as possible as is going to be of use to him in living his life, and to modify the super-ego as far as we possibly can; and to find ways of helping him to reach a capacity for making reparation, because this is something he is going to need to find – and it has got to do with the depressions, of course, because the suicidal bit has partly got to do with the impossibility of making reparation (there are all sorts of other side issues as well). He must feel that what he has done is irretrievable... in fantasy he must have committed many murders, so anything one can do that makes it possible for him to feel that reparation can be reached would help him more than any one other single thing. This will help him to tolerate consciousness of the bit of himself that may remain dangerous to himself and others.

Our aim is to have need assessment files, which will include the whole of the current population of a unit. These will be followed by later assessments, whenever these seem appropriate. We shall then be in a position to consider grouping in terms of emotional compatibility, and to avoid – what happens only too often – the disruption of an integrated group through the presence of a couple of 'frozen' ones, who are not only unable to get help themselves in this setting, but who will make it impossible for others to be helped.

I am well aware that there is a time factor involved, and that, as a consultant, my discussion groups with staff are built into the framework of the organization. Nevertheless, I cannot feel that these are the only circumstances in which need assessments can be made; and indeed, groups working under the leadership of the head of the house have been able to produce excellent assessments. All the same, I incline to the view that every residential unit should have consultancy available to help and support staff in their difficult task. I would suppose that one of these days there will be a training for consultancy in residential work, for which many social workers would be suitable candidates–but that is another story!

It would seem that in undertaking the task of assessment, no one person should be asked to do this alone; and that assessors, avoiding omnipotence in themselves, should not drift into collusion with the omnipotence of others as a means of escape from an intolerable load of responsibility.

10
Consultancy, 1971

This paper was written for an international seminar on consultancy in social work, held at York University in the summer of 1971.

Many years ago something happened to me which I have not forgotten. We were trying at that time to help a small delinquent character in the Mulberry Bush, who was known as Goblin. He had red hair, a bright pink face and a squint. He was goblin-shaped and very slightly spastic. I was talking about him with the psychiatrist who was supervising his treatment with us, Dr Barbara Woodhead, who is a psychoanalyst, one of the consultants who have done most to help the Bush, and to whom I personally am much indebted. Describing Goblin's behaviour, I spoke of his special song, 'Boiled beef and carrots'. He would ask in any situation, 'Would you like a song?', and there would inevitably follow 'Boiled beef and carrots'. Dr Woodhead laughed a little when I told her this, and remarked, 'He's really singing about himself, isn't he?—he *is* boiled beef and carrots, with that carroty hair and his red face!' For a moment I was stunned by a complicated feeling inside me, which I presently recognized as a mixture of envy and anger: envy that Dr Woodhead had understood something which I had missed—anger that I had failed to realize something so evident—evident as soon as she had pointed it out to me!

Recently something else happened to me which I found myself linking with this experience. I was talking with a small girl in a therapeutic school: we had been playing 'squiggles' (Winnicott's technique), and arising from her third squiggle she reached, and communicated, a terrible realization concerned with the beginning of her life (what Sechehaye would term 'symbolic realization'). Julia spoke loudly as her deep feelings burst their bonds and emerged in symbolic description. Now and then she paused for my response: since the meaning of the material was crystal clear, I could make statements based on the child's communications which were valid to her. During this dialogue there must have been a knock on my door which Julia and I were too absorbed to register: when presently she rose to go, we found a student waiting on the landing outside my room. Julia went her way, deep inside herself, and I apologized to the student—I had kept her waiting for several minutes. She came in, sat down, and there was silence for an instant. Then she said abruptly 'I have been eavesdropping... I heard what Julia and you were saying to each other. I want you to know now that I have *never* believed what you have written and said—I have never believed a word! Now, because I listened (I *did* knock, but you didn't hear) I know that children *can* talk like this . . . that these things really happen.' She was very upset, but at the same time she experienced relief: she was actually communicating her envy of me—just the same kind of envy which I had experienced towards Dr Woodhead (and towards many other people who have known and understood more than I could myself).

These two episodes seem to me to typify the core of the consultant's problem—how to help and teach clients, without arousing conscious or unconscious envy, so intolerable that clients may be unable to make use of the help or the teaching, however valid and valuable this may be.

There has been much written about consultancy, although not enough concerning consultancy in residential work. Kaplan, Bettelheim and others have made important contributions on this subject: my own task in this paper is—as I have stated in my title—to describe my personal experience as a consultant, and also as one who has made use of available consultancy, especially in the residential treatment of severely deprived and unintegrated children and adolescents. It may well be that other workers will have had very different experiences, which they will realize and communicate in their own personal mode. This need not invalidate their work or my own. It is important to establish at once that I am writing (and usually do write) from a subjective standpoint—personal and special, rather than impersonal and general—although possibly we may be able to reach some general conclusions, such as my threshold statement that *envy is a factor which cannot be ignored in consultancy*. My aim is to share my own experiences with you, in the hope that by considering these, and conceptualizations based on actual work, we may be able to pinpoint the difficulties of consultancy in residential work and make some suggestions with regard to a hypothetical training in residential consultancy.

I have found through work over many years in residential places that in common with others I can be of far more use to children if I work through the staff, rather than attempt direct treatment by psychotherapy myself. This way of working does not preclude occasional 'key' sessions with children, either at their request or that of the worker involved (under no circumstances would I work with a child against his will). Now and then the child may need a brief series of such key sessions, usually at some crisis in evolvement. In the main, however, my discussions with staff members seem more appropriate to a situation in which the workers are in reality the therapists. My own role thus becomes supportive to the conscious involvements which are an essential part in the providing of primary experience. There is a grave danger that people working in a place can attribute to a consultant magical and omniscient powers, so that, relieved of responsibility, they can refer a child to the consultant, feeling thereafter that treatment is now 'out of their hands': at the same time, should the child act out or develop symptoms, they are likely to attribute such manifestations to the work of the psychotherapist. From the start, in working with a staff group I have found it essential to establish my own role as being supportive to the therapists in the place in *their* work with children. This role can be frustrating, and I have always had private patients of my own elsewhere, in order to enable me to tolerate working 'once removed' from children in residential places. The children themselves seem to reach a clear understanding about my contribution to the work of the place— even asking for certain problems to be discussed with me.

I was recently asked for a brief internal report on my task as a consultant at the Cotswold Community. In quoting from this, I hope to give some idea of the type of work needed in this field of residential work. The Cotswold Community used to be a rigid approved school, which over the past four years has been changed into a therapeutic community, under the directorship of Richard Balbernie.

MY TASK AS CONSULTANT AT THE COTSWOLD COMMUNITY

Initially, we saw my tasks to be (firstly) the provision of ego

support in order to facilitate ego functioning in integrated children; (secondly) the containment of unintegrated children with
provision of primary experience with which to build the self and
achieve integration. These two tasks were to be carried out
through work with both staff and boys. It was assumed that
unintegrated children would form a small minority group in the
place: this group would need, as soon as possible, to be insulated
in order to receive appropriate treatment. The mixture of integrated and unintegrated boys was recognized as undesirable.

In the event, I was assigned to a house (St David's) consisting
of very deprived and disturbed boys: this group was not yet
separated in any way from the rest of the Community, but was
self-selective in terms of gross disturbance as a common factor.
I talked with the boys and with the staff invidually, until the staff
themselves asked for group meetings with me. These staff groups
became the nucleus of my work in the Community. My sessions
with boys could—with their permission—be used to help staff to
gain insight and to understand the need for teamwork in order
to provide experience. These individual sessions were—and remain
—of necessity brief (twenty to thirty minutes). I have found that
where residential workers are themselves carrying out a therapeutic programme, sessions with individual boys have what I call
a 'key' function, helping to open and deepen channels of communication between boys and workers.

St David s became presently the unit for unintegrated boys
known as 'the Cottage'. Once this kind of insulation had been
established, my task became more precise. By discussing weekly
'happenings' chosen by the Cottage team, I was able to help them
to provide primary experience through individual adaptation to
need, based on an early kind of dependence and involving localized regression within a relationship in a firmly structured containing environment. In this way, the team came to realize how
disciplined any real therapeutic work must be, and the danger of
collusion and the need for confrontation of a non-punitive kind.
The team did good work, although naturally making many mistakes which with adequate support they could face. The development of an ego culture in the Cottage minimized authoritarian
attitudes at one extreme, and subcultures at the other. The establishment of open communication between staff and boys reduced

acting out; and the insulation and containment of this group of unintegrated boys enabled ego growth and strengthening in other groups within the Community.

For various reasons it was decided after a time that I should work in a similar consultant-tutor role in the remaining three house teams. My weekly discussion groups evolved into seminars, with learning based on the group experiences during the current week. Each group seminar lasts for forty-five minutes, with periods of from twenty to thirty minutes available (as before) for key sessions with boys (usually at their own request) and tutorials with team members–often the heads of houses. There is also a new housemothers' group. I have a close liaison with Trevor Blewett, the head of group living, who plans my day's work each week, and with whom I discuss my work in detail each Wednesday evening on the telephone, after my return home. I also have meetings with Mike Jinks, head of education. I meet Richard Balbernie, the Principal, frequently, and discuss problems and recommendations with him, both at the Cotswold and by telephone.

The development of a system of need assessment has enabled me to chart all houses on a basis of integrated or unintegrated: and if unintegrated, to chart the specific syndrome of deprivation (see chapters 8 and 9). From this 'inside diagnosis' we are now in a position to plan treatment on a basis of need, and to select with some certainty those boys to whom we can offer help. The work on need assessment is also enabling the staff to conceptualize and communicate what they are doing; and recently teams have begun to carry out these assessments themselves, checking results with me, so that we can plan treatment programmes in an exact way.

We hope to establish a plan for intake, which will exclude the occasional case which we cannot contain (a boy with a considerable psychotic pocket). Interviewing boys whose suitability is in doubt also comes into my task area.

This way of working brings me into contact with most people working in the Community, and enables me consequently to consider the total state of the place at any time. I am also in a position from which it is feasible to support the primary tasks in any group situation: at the same time recognizing and stopping what I have come to think of as the 'anti-tasks' which exist in every residential place, and which involve a collusive undertow of subculture (including adults and boys), undermining the ego functioning of the group and wrecking the primary task. The fact that there is a large proportion of unintegrated boys in the total group, a much larger proportion than we imagined originally, makes the presence of anti-task a constant hazard. I think that the fact I really respect the house teams, expecting them to carry out therapy themselves, helps them to accept my contribution to their increasingly skilled work.

TASK AND ANTI-TASK

The treatment of severely emotionally deprived children must take place in the context of what is happening in this place at this moment with this person (because unintegrated children have no realization of past or future). It is useless to confront a delinquent, for example, in retrospect; one must be *there* in the situation, anticipating acting out by the provision of communication. The consultant is of no use next day or next week—not even a few hours later—what is necessary is that the people in the place should have (or gain) the necessary skills and insight to carry out the work themselves.

The climate of a therapeutic school must always produce at least elements of a crisis culture—emotionally deprived children tend to live from crisis to crisis. The survival of such a place is often in question for obvious reasons. This leads to a paranoid position in which the grown-ups in the place—the treatment team—present a united front which is dependent on hostile outsiders to maintain the unity. The fact that there are really enemies, and others who say 'We are on your side', tends to perpetuate this unhappy state of affairs. A crisis culture of this sort is likely to breed anti-task, springing from those elements in children, staff and management which are unconsciously ranged against primary task.

I think there must always be anti-task present to some degree: the safety and survival of primary task is dependent upon enough ability and security to confront anti-task. If anti-task is not confronted, collusive anxiety can lead to states of panic, immobilization, and breakdown.

It is from anti-task activity that subculture grows, and there must always be some risks of this destructive phenomenon coming into being. The more secure the team groups, the smaller the risk, because confrontation of anti-task and subculture becomes felt as less dangerous. I think that collusive anxiety and collusion itself are great hazards in all residential work–including consultancy.

In a residential place, one often finds what I think of as a 'fallacy of a delusional equilibrium', maintained through collusive anxiety, so that anti-task may be covered, as it were, by a thin sheet of ice on which the people of the place skate at hazard.

The surfacing of anti-task is always painful, but the maintenance of a delusional equilibrium is self-destructive. It is better to have our feet on solid ground–however rocky–than to fear ice cracking beneath us. I find that supporting a team in the surfacing and confronting of anti-task can be a service which can strengthen the group ego.

In my report on my task in the Cotswold Community, I referred to 'need assessments'. The use of this kind of technique seems to me to be essential in focusing, as it does, the attention of the whole group (including the consultant) on the primary task–in our case, the provision of primary experience. On the basis that anti-task, acting out, and subcultures of all kinds tend to spring from a breakdown in real communication, it would seem of the utmost importance to keep all lines of communication open– between members of the team, between grown-ups and children, and between the consultant and all others in the place. The making of a need assessment involves the whole staff group of a residential unit, working with the consultant, and pooling resources in order to evaluate need.

Often insights are reached in the making of these assessments which are not only of value to the child under consideration, but also the treatment team themselves, throwing light on problems of delusional counter-transference–splitting mechanisms, for example–but in a way which is tolerable because it is indirect and shared. Such an approach seems to me to give child care workers a proper professional position in the scheme of things–the consultant being entirely dependent on the material brought forward by the unit team (see chapters 8 & 9).

In the need assessment questions I have used the terms to which

I am accustomed, giving explanations. In this way the workers involved have become used to distinctions such as 'empathy' compared with 'projective identification', 'personal guilt' (concern) as compared with 'fear of revenge' (talion guilt), and so on. At first, the going is slow and the reporting scant. Very soon, however, the task draws out the group potential. There is plenty of opportunity for argument and doubt. I find myself more easily accepted than in other forms of group reporting. As a result of discussing concepts such as 'merger', 'psychotic pocket' or 'burnt-out autism', workers wish to read papers and to reach further conceptualization, *because* this reaching out for more is based on their own experiences and realizations (I only provide ways of communicating these). The problem of envy of the consultant is much less likely to turn up, because anything that I can offer is at their disposal: I am not in a defended position. The need assessment which follows is on a small boy (aged seven) who has recently come to the Bush: this is a first assessment.

CHRISTOPHER'S NEED ASSESSMENT

I.Q. 100

Disruption. Yes.

Panic. One would certainly get the impression that there is some evidence of panic, but less frequent than when he arrived. He can spiral from an ordinary situation into panic—an area of panic in the total situation. The panic states he gets into are concerned with dependence. He may have used threats of panic state to get what he wants from grown-ups and then simulated panic states: his parents' reaction to this is to act out, and his mother will dissociate herself completely (we saw this happen here when the parents visited).

Classification: Unintegrated.

Guilt, personal concern: There is denial plus apparent outrage at being suspected (this is probably a very intellectual defence).

Dependence, trust: He is looking for the possibility of dependence and wanting to reach it: he is already dependent on Douglas Hawkins (child care worker) and this had grown, due to the hospital situation (i.e. when Christopher broke his leg and was in hospital overnight and most of the second day). When John Armstrong (headmaster) was carrying Christopher he was trusting and really clinging.

Merger: No evidence.

Empathy: None.

Stress: There is verbal and physical aggression. He has a highly developed technique of logical argument; he keeps things under control by this kind of argument. He communicates in a stressful situation (the logical argument is probably a defence).

Communication: Symbolic communication at a fairly deep level— one example was concerned with the period when he was in hospital and away from the school for about twenty-six hours. He communicates more easily in moments of stress. There is non-verbal communication in which he indicates his need quite clearly. There is a little bond which continues with B.D-D.—he appeared at the door of her room at a time when she had someone else there and was not able to give time to Christopher, she explained. He went off, then returned and asked for some paper and a pencil. Since then, from time to time, he comes and is supplied with sheets of paper and a pencil—as yet this situation has not advanced in any way.

Identification: Quite a lot of projective identification—Christopher asked for his clean clothes with the firm intention of getting ready for the arrival of another boy's parents and going out with them (this, of course, was not allowed). He aims at obtaining experience secondhand. He tends to identify with his father: and Christopher does 'switch off', and this could be identification with his mother, who dissociates.

Depression: There is not a depressed mood.

Aggression: Yes, verbal and physical.

Capacity for play: On the whole, his play is narcissistic: he enjoys play with water, paint, sand (he bends the rules, cheats).

Capacity for learning: He presumably does learn from experience— he has got as far as he has by insisting on being taken care of; he has fought for this care by rumpus-raising and any other means that work, and for a while, as long as these methods work for him, he will continue to use them. There are signs that this particular mechanism is declining as he finds his needs are being met (at a mealtime, on being given his milk, he will say 'And fill it right to the top'). There was a little game with B.D-D., when Christopher was in bed, with circus, clowns, masks: B.D-D.

suggested that it might not now be so necessary for Christopher to hide behind a mask–he smiled.

Self preservation: He does get hurt a lot: he cuts himself, falls over (the broken leg now, and various other accidents).

False self. (Comment from B.D.-D.)–A false-self child who will get to regression and deep dependence–probably rather total regression. From the description of him in bed and what I met of him in bed, I would think that the accidents, disasters, illnesses and anything else he can collect of this sort are, in fact, opportunities for regression and that he can then be at peace. One gets the impression that he makes good use of all these things that are happening to him.

One must look for adaptations leading to regression; notice anything he says or indicates about things that are suitable for him –like the cup of milk that has to be filled right up–this is obviously something important to him. Slowly, one hopes, he will establish stepping stones to get his regression, and accidents and goodness knows what, and that seems unnecessary.

He will have to reach considerable ego strength to be able to cope with his parents–even assuming they do remain together.

Such a child can arouse much hostility in a treatment unit because of his initial *un*dependence; his apparent ability to do without us is a threat to people who want to be of use to deprived children.

The team at the Bush have considerable insight, and can comment on their own defences, and to some extent clear them out of the way. The shared experience of the need assessment helps the team and myself to orientate more directly and simply to the now defined task, to provide a regression for Christopher, with stepping stones of adaptation: for example, the paper and pencil, the full cup of milk, and the symbolic communication. The special kind of reliability which he is meeting from everyone (especially from Douglas) will lead him to put down further stepping stones towards regression. The regression itself may well be managed by several people who will support each other in order to ensure continuity of care and symbolic provision. My main task will be to support the team and to share realizations with them as we go along together. This kind of support really has much in common with that needed by 'the ordinary devoted mother', the difference being that this is conscious and professional work, where intuition is not enough.

CONCLUSION

As a consultant in residential work, I find that my own considerable experience of working as an 'insider'—a therapist *in* a therapeutic community—is invaluable, now that I work as an outsider coming into the place. My analysis, and the tremendous help I have received myself from consultants, help me to empathize with others in consultancy with me. Finally, my conviction that therapy in a residential place must be carried out by the people in the place helps to avoid a 'we' and 'they' situation, in which massive defences and counter-defences can cripple open communication between consultant and treatment team.

I I

The management of violence
in disturbed children, 1971

This paper was read late in 1970 *as my contribution to a seminar on violence run by the Department of Health and Social Security. The material at the end of the paper was an experiment for use in discussion groups, and was sufficiently successful for me to wish to repeat the technique.*

An outbreak of violence in any human being, grown-up or child, is always frightening to a degree, because we know, consciously or intuitively, that here is the expression of feelings so terrible as not to be containable. We are sometimes conscious of violence in ourselves which we cannot always successfully contain, but which most of the time is deep in our unconscious: potential, but untapped. The explosion of another's violence reminds us of this potential in ourselves, perhaps of occasions when even to some much lesser extent our own violence has come into our consciousness and may have to some degree been acted out in our environment.

During the first year of life, babies change from being contained (by their mothers and the holding environment) to becoming 'containers'. There are no feelings stronger, deeper, or more overwhelming than those which are already experienced at this early date. The 'ordinary devoted mother' (Winnicott) can contain the baby's rage and her own feelings as long as this is necessary – until the baby can contain his own feelings. Many of the children in our care have not become containers: at five, ten or fifteen years they may still need a lot of containment in order to integrate into whole, containing people. In the meantime, they are liable to act out their intolerably violent emotions in many ways, damaging to other people, themselves and their environment.

Winnicott defined panic as 'unthinkable anxiety'. Much violence is caused by panic states: *thinking* is an essential way of containing feelings. Communication of such thoughts to others can be an unknown safety valve – if the thoughts are not there, they cannot be communicated; the anxiety is then so terrible and primitive as to be unthinkable, and the child reaches a panic state in which he may be totally immobilized, or dreadfully active.

One could say that the communication of violent feelings in words to another person is a symbolic way of finding a person able and willing to contain the child and his feelings.

A neurotic, integrated child (i.e. a well-established 'container', with boundaries to himself and an inner reality within him) will be able to make such communication if it can reach consciousness. An integrated child has many means at his disposal of containing terrible feelings. For example, he can repress his violent aggression, or he can convert this into a symptom, or he can sublimate the aggression, putting it to some useful purpose. Usually a neurotic, integrated child will only experience the occasional twinge of panic with which we are all familiar; he is only likely to explode briefly and in a localized way into violence, and is usually able to put his feelings into words—even though these may be screamed.

The deprived, unintegrated child has no such resources. Where the integrated can *respond* to crisis, the unintegrated *reacts* to what he feels to be the threat of total annihilation. For him, conflict is not the question, but rather survival, not only of himself but of *everything*. Annihilation of the kind I am describing is something comparable to 'the end of the world'. Even integrated people can experience this dread now and then, but they are not constantly exposed to the threat of infinite destruction, in the way that deprived and unintegrated children seem to be; nor do they have to manage annihilating forces within themselves. Unintegrated people simply *overflow* into violence: integrated people disintegrate into areas of violence—they are much less at risk than the former group.

At the present time, groups in residential places are a mixture of integrated and unintegrated—this demands tolerance of a high degree of incompatibility by children and staff: I have written elsewhere about this (see chapter 3), and would draw your attention to this aspect of the film *John*[1], in which an integrated toddler was exposed to the full blast of unintegrated peers, with appalling

---

[1] See note to page 72.

results. There would perhaps be less disastrous effects of separation if the dangers of incompatible mixing were more generally recognized.

In any community home there are likely to be several unintegrated, uncontaining children who are certain to break down into violence which will harm others and themselves. Unintegrated children are not especially disturbed by these explosions which come into their 'scene'. Integrated children are terribly threatened by violence because they *can disintegrate*, which unintegrated ones cannot do because they have never been 'in one piece' and are not whole people.

The grown-ups involved in such a situation are also frightened and disturbed, and this can affect them in all sorts of ways, depending on individual personalities. Institutionalization and hierarchical management are defences against these fears. Workers may 'switch off' feelings, depersonalize, become cold and pseudo-objective, and hand over the 'happening' to superiors, or become violent themselves.

Descriptions of violent behaviour in children tend to be detached, in a way which leaves the grown-up in a superior position. The grown-up may become 'angry' and the child has a 'temper tantrum'. The grown-up asserts, in such a context, that the violence is that of childhood–there is a deep unwillingness to face the fact that grown-ups are not so different in reality, and are also capable of having temper tantrums . It is difficult for a grown-up to admit that he has behaved violently towards a child, because he feels himself to be too mature for such behaviour. Really it becomes essential for the person working with children to be well aware of the possible violence within himself. We all know the gentle, patient person who arranges (unconsciously, of course) for children to act out his violence while he stays calm and 'good'.

'Punishment' is often a rationalization of violence–grown-ups can act out, denying the real causes within themselves which lead to their violent actions.

If one can see all acting out as a breakdown in communication –an area in which the individual cannot contain and think about his feelings, then one's attitude is more honest and less defended, so that one is actually more free to take appropriate action and to make comments which are valuable to the child.

Thinking about children and violence, I find myself considering two phases: (1) before the violent act takes place, and (2) after the act of violence has been committed. Anticipation of violence calls for good observation, empathy, and a feeling for dynamics – 'one thing leads to another'. Too often 'another' has been reached without 'one thing' having been observed and registered.

Panic states are, in a sense, psychosomatic. One can observe physical symptoms in a child one has come to know. Pallor, trembling, change of voice and breathing, dilation of the eyes, and a desperate restlessness may all be signals of an approaching storm. At this stage, insulation and containment may save the child and the environment from disaster. There was much to criticize in the film '*Warrendale*'[1], but here at least an effort was made to contain the child and his feelings *in time*. The point is often made that 'nothing has happened to cause the outbursts of violence'. The truth is that we may not have realized what has happened to the child in terms of his inner reality. *Something*–a look, a word, a circumstance, may have set up a chain of associations which will have forced him to remember through feeling 'other voices, other rooms' (Capote).

Emotionally deprived children are traumatized at a stage so early that they cannot realize, symbolize or conceptualize what has happened to them: they 'remember' only through feeling. *There is no way of containing traumata*. This is how I understand the aetiology of panic states and the violence which springs from them.

Panic is contagious: adults, even experienced workers, can catch panic from children. This contagious quality is generally recognized in crowd panics (football disasters, fires in cinemas or theatres, for example) but is less easily seen in individual panic states. This infection partly explains the immobilization which can beset grown-ups confronted by violence. One has to hold on to one's identity, to guard the frontiers of one's self in a situation. To *contain* the child and his violence is not the same as to merge with him.

There is a tendency to identify with violence in a very primitive and unconscious way. I knew a family once–all grown up–which contained a schizophrenic brother, hospitalized from time to

[1] '*Warrendale*', Allan King, 1967.

time, but for the most part living at home and causing chaos. An elder brother who owned a shop had just installed a large plateglass show window; the schizophrenic one, in a moment of rage, smashed the new plateglass window to smithereens. When the family told me of this disaster, there was unmistakeable envy in their voices—envy of the ill brother who could do this terrible, violent act and 'get away with it'!

Often, in the therapeutic institutions where I work, children have said to me 'I really don't know how I came to do it' in describing some act of violence. But often, going carefully over the events of that day, we have been able to find a terrible build-up of unnoticed tension, leading to final breakdown. The child may even have been actually conscious of the tension and its causes, but there has been no opportunity to communicate this to a grown up in time. So here the child and I are, in retrospect, trying to talk about what should have been in the future and is now in the past.

A boy, Tom, aged nine, at the Mulberry Bush some years ago broke windows for no apparent cause, and with tremendous violence. It was finally possible to link these explosions with a breakdown in communication with his mother. When this happened—when no letter arrived—Tom became convinced that she was dead. Waiting for the news of her death produced tension and panic so terrific that the smashing of glass produced temporary relief.

I have spoken of moments of panic violence in integrated children, and of prolonged panic states leading to violence in unintegrated ones: there is another more rare category of violence, but one which I suspect is more common than one would suppose. This is the violence displayed by a more or less integrated child who has a psychotic pocket. This pocket of madness is not emotionally linked to the rest of him: he has integrated 'round a hole'. This means in effect that he can suddenly depart, as it were, into the mad bit of himself, so that an apparently well-behaved, sensible boy can suddenly commit violent crimes; and having done so, return into the major, sane part of himself. The mad bit is hidden from himself, as it is from others, although there are unmistakeable clues as to the presence of the psychotic pocket.

We are concerned here today with all these kinds of violence, whatever form they may take, as we meet children's outbursts in residential treatment. All violence has a quality of orgasm: it is preceded by an intense spiral of excitement, leading to climax and followed by relief and subsidence. Panic is, at its climax, a kind of traumatic orgasm. Violent behaviour has always sexual undertones, sometimes conscious ones. The sexuality can, however, range from displaced infantile greed (delinquency) to genital sexuality (rape). There are often particular fantasies which accompany the violent behaviour. Essentially, however, I believe that children are swept along by violence: they can do terrible things in cold blood, but these are usually sadistic and not necessarily *violent*. Violence, as I understand the phenomenon, implies a loss of control, a helpless rage.

The management of violence, as I have indicated earlier in this paper, has two phases. Ideally, there should be anticipation, so that the violent act does not have to take place. Failing anticipation, there must be containment and control of the violent out-of-control child in a panic. Essential at both stages is communication: although the child does not seem to hear a word one is saying at the time, he will remind one, years later, of communications made in such circumstances. All acting out is broken down communication, and we can build a bridge even in a welter of flailing legs and arms, gnashing teeth, spitting mouth, and snarling, shrieking voice. *If you can communicate, he can hear.* What one communicates depends on each individual child and the context, but there are basic assumptions which we can start from – the child's helplessness, the echo of early trauma, the helpless infantile rage (however big he may be). So that, for example, when a boy yells 'Leave me alone' it is appropriate to reply 'I promise not to leave you.' The most valuable thing we can do in such circumstances is to continue to be alive, reliable and concerned. I always hold on when a child is in a panic state: I hold his hand, trying not to lose my hold, and I continue to communicate. I may have an arm round the child. We may be standing or sitting; he may be lying on his back, or whirling around me; but I try to hold on, and if I do lose my hold on his hand I re-establish this as soon as I can. This is not so difficult, because part of him *wants* to be held. Presently, he will be the one who is doing the holding, and the worst is then over.

Anticipation very often *precipitates* the panic state: but we are then in a position of strength to hold the child and his rage, and to prevent the violent act which would have followed. Really, every act of violence which we have to consider in retrospect is basically a failure in management.

Bruno Bettelheim, in his book *The Children of the Dream* concerning Kibbutzim, which some of you may have read, writes:

> Conversely, being sure of one's place might explain another striking contrast to what is typical in our society, and why kibbutz childhood is such a happy age. Not once did I observe any physical fighting among kibbutz children. Not once—beyond the age when they push each other down in the playpen—did I see a child pushing another, not to mention hitting with hand or object. This does not occur in the kibbutz. I asked about it repeatedly, and the answer was always the same; while there are disagreements, they never go beyond verbal expression. There are no fights about things like who comes first, or who sits where. Compared with the frequent fighting that seems typical in our society among pre-school and grammar-school children, life in the kibbutz at this age is peaceful indeed.
>
> Of course, it helps that there are no possessions to fight over and no social distinctions. But much of the fighting at this age in our society originates in the child's feeling that he has no place that is rightfully his. He must fight first to assert it and then to maintain it—whether the unending fight explodes in physical violence, or is carried on in more hidden form.

Here we might pause to consider Robert Ardry's 'Territorial Imperative', which in human beings means basically 'room'—emotional and physical—in which to be an individual. Very often this is *not* available to severely deprived children. On the other hand, the idealized institutionalization which dominates a kibbutz denies the child the right to be an individual.

In this connection it seems important to consider what Winnicott wrote about depression.

> The main thing is that depression indicates that the individual is accepting responsibility for the aggressive and destructive elements in human nature. This means that the depressed person has a capacity for holding a certain amount of guilt (about matters that are chiefly unconscious), and this allows of a sear-

ching round for an opportunity for constructive activity.

Our violent deprived children have not reached this position. I have spoken of containers; destructive feelings and guilt must be contained if the person is to have a real identity.

I want now to consider the actual presence of violence and how we can manage the child and his violence in a therapeutic and non-punitive or retaliatory way. I assume this is the problem for all of us: we may understand the causes of violence, but how do we actually deal with violent behaviour?

Some years ago James, a ten-year-old, was provoked by a younger boy, on whom he then made what was really a murderous attack; if he could have killed the younger boy he would have done so. Intervention took place instantly, but we had not been quick enough to anticipate disaster. I spent the next hour trying to keep in touch, physically and emotionally, with James, who was tied up in knots on his bed, shrieking obscenities (the violence had taken place in a dormitory). I kept on talking: about James, his pain and anguish, his intolerable panic state. He did not seem to register what I was saying until suddenly he screamed at me, 'People like you don't understand people like me—I've murdered love!' He felt that he had destroyed everything.

Another boy aged thirteen, who was very tall and strong, took up a large lump of coal and threw it at my head—he was only a few yards away. I could see that he was going to do this, but there was no one near enough to intervene: so I froze in my tracks and the coal whistled past my ear. A moment later he was stumbling over to me, white and crying. He said, 'I've always known I'd have to try and kill you.' His mother had left him and his father.

There was a ten-year-old, Jeremy, who was epileptic and very disturbed. When he first came to us from a mental hospital, he would stand in the middle of his bed, swinging a full hotwater bottle round his head, and shrieking, 'I'm going to throw it at you'. I used to stand at the end of the bed, talking to him, and ultimately he would burst into tears, throwing the hot bottle on to the floor. His parents had been terrified of him. In this case holding was not necessary.

Peter used to hit people—children and grown-ups—with all his strength: this was so sudden as to be impossible to anticipate.

He was a large tough thirteen-year-old. We discovered that he could not believe that he could *reach* anyone: the blow was a distorted communication. Interpretation brought him enough trust to reach out to others.

Compare these outbursts of violence with the case of a small patient of mine, Edward, aged four, who described the monsters in the garden who threatened him at night. These were his own uncontainable violent feelings, projected on to his environment. It is true that Edward did not commit violent acts, but neither (at that time) could he contain these terrible feelings. He became threatened by them from outside himself; he took up a paranoid position, living in anguish and fear.

All these children were unintegrated: the violence of integrated people is much more localized–in fact they partially *disintegrate* into violence. The more integrated the person, the quicker and easier will it be to re-establish thinking and communication, thereby enabling the child to *complete the experience*. I think that the concept of the complete experience is important in this connection. Nightmares are usually interrupted dreams–the dreamer can find no solution, so he wakes. In the same way the child can feel unable to resolve some intolerable situation: he tries to 'wake up', to escape from the terrible stress, but he *is* awake, so he collapses into panic. As I have said earlier, this can take the form of violence or immobilization, even the loss of consciousness.

In all these examples I have given there has been a breakdown in communication: the restoration of thinking in words restores stability, and makes the dangerous feelings containable. It is an awful fact that well-meaning people can provoke violence by irrelevant and inappropriate value judgments. For example, a child desperately trying to reach communication with a grown-up may be termed 'attention seeking'. When *we* ask someone 'Are you paying attention?' we mean 'Are you listening?' Of course children need, and ask for, our attention: what they are saying is urgent. Equally, when an infuriated youngster shouts an answer to some accusation or criticism, he may well be told not to 'answer back'. I have never been able to understand this ridiculous phrase. This kind of grown-up behaviour can trigger off violence in every form: people are shutting off the safety-valve of speech. Perhaps one of the problems lies in the fact that one tends to understand

what a child is saying (or what he is likely to say) in such circumstances to be an accusation. If, instead of accusing us, he attacks
someone else, or smashes the place to smithereens, or sets fire
to a barn, *we do not have to understand* what he might have said.
We can just be angry with him for what he has done, and get rid
of our own feelings of guilt.

Actually, the establishment of communication with disturbed
children always leads to a torrent of accusation in the first place,
directed against ourselves and everyone else. It is essential in
therapeutic work to be able to accept the reality of the *feelings*
expressed, and not to waste time arguing about the facts, which
are probably quite otherwise but are in any case irrelevant.

How one responds to violence or to communication of violent
feelings depends on the kind of person one happens to be. One
person may say 'How can you talk about your mother like this?'
when in reality the grown-up would like to say some pretty awful
things about his own mother but is not in a position to do so.
Or he can say 'But you *know* Miss A is always so kind to you . . . '
when everyone knows that Miss A does not get on at all well
with this particular child.

A terrifying fact is that behaviour can be interpreted incorrectly
as violent, and such interpretation can be accepted by the child
on to whom it is projected. A boy in a residential place met a staff
wife out walking with her dog. She was carrying a chain lead.
She did not know Johnnie, who had just arrived, but greeted him.
He trailed along behind her, making vague remarks; he asked to
carry the chain, which she gave to him. He walked on, swinging
the chain, and presently he said that he wanted to show her a
damaged puppy nearby. She followed him, but there was no
puppy. She asked him for the chain, which he gave to her, and
then he took off his jersey, twisted it, and swung this instead of
the chain 'as though it were a rope'. There were various myths
concerned with violence and this boy, and when this episode was
reported to me there was the implication that violence was present
just below the surface. In fact, the 'damaged puppy' represented
Johnnie himself; the chain or lead and the 'rope' of jersey were
links to a grown-up, a seeking for dependence, in a strange place
(I knew enough about Johnnie to be sure of this). If Johnnie had
collected this projection (he did not) he could have *felt* that he

was a violent person.

On rare occasions a woman may be really threatened by a violent boy in a residential place. He may need to be physically controlled for her safety and his own. Whenever possible she should call for help from a man, rather than involve herself in physical struggle with the child. Nothing is more disastrous than for a woman to lose her role and act like a man, using her strength to overcome a boy. Some women seem to need to show how physically strong they are, but in doing so they lose their emotional strength (in the same way it is sad when a mother has to be a father to her son).

Men may use much more strength than is necessary in order to control a violent child: perhaps because they assert their masculine power which is threatened; perhaps because there are homosexual elements present, although unconscious. In the same way, women can be sexually aroused by a struggle with a violent boy or girl. Because this is unconscious they may provoke this sort of battle in order to obtain sexual excitement. Really it is very seldom necessary to use physical force, although holding a child firmly with one's arm round him, or holding his hand, may be very necessary. To react to violence with violence is only likely to promote more violence: there is a narrow margin between 'strength' and 'violence'.

There is also what I think of as 'institutionalized violence', the extreme versions of which are execution and killing in battle. Here, violent acts are rationalized by organization and hierarchy. One sees this in the use of violence in punishment. Such acts— beating, for example—are organized with great care, with respect for hierarchy, rules and ceremonies: in this way the face of violence is masked. In Ireland in the eighteenth century the hangman wore a horrific animal mask in order to hide his identity from society.

I have been in institutions where there is excellent order and control, reasonably benign authority, and no sign of violence in management of children. On the other hand, the children seem too quiet, too passive: on further investigation I have found that in such a place the newcomer is exposed to violent treatment so that he becomes afraid. There is then no need for more than threat —discipline and control can be easily maintained. One is reminded of a disturbed small child who shows one a fly which he has already half stunned, saying, 'Look how tame it is—it doesn't want to leave me.' Of course there is a lot of collusion involved in such a state of affairs: people are often thankful to wear blinkers.

Gang violence in a place has much in common with this kind of institutionalized violence. Children in a delinquent group in a subculture will also commit violent acts (under cover of 'initiation', for example). The leader of such a gang is liable to have a psychotic pocket. Subcultures flourish in a punitive climate in which violence is implicit when not explicit. Some people assume that this kind of subculture is 'part of the scene'. This is not a valid assumption: lack of communication between staff and children can lead to the first signs of subculture. There is no reason why such a growth should flourish unless there is collusive anxiety present in the adult group (who will have a subculture of their own). Confrontation, recognition of the 'storm centre'—the delinquent hero—and establishment of real communication, will remove the need for the subculture; which, in a group, is rather like autism in an individual.

When a grown-up hits a child in a moment of rage, this is a violent act which must never be denied. Nobody ought to strike a child, but if this happens the fact should be communicated to others, and the child should understand clearly that the grown-up has been unable to control or contain his anger. Certainly a blow in anger is preferable to a planned beating, because we are not deceiving the child or ourselves in the former circumstances.

You will have noticed that I have drifted over a wide field in this chapter. The point is that this *is* a large field; violence is as it were the infra-red of every spectrum. The possibility of violence is always implicit in every situation that involves people in relation to one another, because violence is there in all of us. The more conscious we can be of our own potential violence, the less likely are we to become violent ourselves, and the more able shall we be to understand and manage violence in others when this is necessary.

AN EPISODE OF VIOLENCE

Henry, aged eight, was a very disturbed boy of high intelligence, placed in a residential special school for maladjusted children. This was the first day of the summer term. His mother had brought him on the afternoon before to the station to meet staff from the school, who had come to London to bring children back to the school in —— shire: Henry and his mother had arrived just in time to catch the train.

The night before, Henry had overheard a terrible outburst of anger between his parents, during which his father had threatened once again to leave him and his mother. His mother had spoken softly, and he could only hear the murmur of her voice going on and on.

After returning to the school, there had not been a suitable moment for Henry to speak about his anxiety to a 'special' grown-up because of the general rush of settling down in the school. The child care worker to whom he would have communicated his anxiety as he had done in the past was on leave. This worker was kind and gentle: she always listened intently, was appalled by his father's outbursts and deeply sorry for his mother—it comforted Henry to talk to her. When Henry's mother came to the school, Mary, this worker, would listen to her complaints about her husband with deep sympathy. Henry's father rarely visited the school: Mary did not talk with him in her soft, quiet voice—she could not bear to do so.

On the morning in question, Henry was no longer thinking about his worry, but was chatting to other children and to the child care staff, who were helping them to get dressed. One of the children said 'I wonder if it's going to rain ...' and Henry said 'Of course not, look how blue the sky is' (there were quite a few dark clouds). He was not hungry at breakfast. At assembly, the children said the Lord's Prayer: towards the end, Henry stopped saying the well-known words, and did not even think them inside himself. Later, his teacher, who was a man whom Henry knew and liked well, asked the children to write an essay about 'My Holidays'. Suddenly the whole horror of the situation at home came back into his mind: he sat, staring in front of him, and was startled when the teacher asked him 'What's wrong?' Henry started to write 'I went to the zoo ...' At lunch time, he still was not hungry. He felt awfully full, stuffed, it was as though something was choking him. People asked him if he was ill, but he shook his head. Anything said to him now seemed like a blow, which made him wince, and any contact became intolerable. He no longer knew what was causing him such anguish which seemed to engulf him. He went out after lunch into the playground in a daze.

Suddenly another boy punched him in the back. This was not a hard punch, but Henry felt a burning behind his nose; he shivered all over and turned white. In an instant, he had thrown himself screaming on the other boy, knocked him down, and tried to strangle him. Staff intervened, and with difficulty pulled Henry away from the boy he was attacking and held him while he screamed and kicked. They tried to understand what had gone wrong, but he was too distressed to speak or even think. He was put to bed for the rest of the day. On the following morning he got up as usual....

Index